Anorexic bodies

A striking example of a 'woman's' illness, anorexia nervosa has previously been studied in isolation from history and politics. *Anorexic Bodies* explores a set of complex theories which together explain anorexia more adequately. The book examines the premise that the body is a 'concept' rather than a simple physical organism and it demonstrates how gender divisions are reflected in current understandings of the body by studying access to women's bodies in rape and representations of women's bodies in pornography. *Anorexic Bodies* uses original interview material to demonstrate a sociological and feminist understanding of the construction of women's bodies in anorexia.

Anorexia is treated as 'an extended example' of how women both resist and are constrained by the cultural concept of the female body. Anorexia is examined as a strategy of resistance, which ultimately becomes its own prison. For it seeks to do individually what can only be done collectively – to challenge the construction and control of women's bodies.

Morag MacSween is a feminist sociologist and currently co-ordinates the Manchester Survivors' Project.

First published 1993
by Routledge
11 New Fetter Lane, London EC4P 4EE

Simultaneously published in the USA and Canada
by Routledge
29 West 35th Street, New York, NY 10001

First published in paperback 1995

Reprinted 1996

Typeset in Baskerville by Michael Mepham, Frome, Somerset
Printed and bound in Great Britain by
T. J. Press (Padstow) Ltd, Padstow, Cornwall

British Library Cataloguing in Publication Data
A catalogue record for this book is available from the British
Library

Library of Congress Cataloguing in Publication Data
A catalogue record for this book is available from the Library of
Congress

ISBN 0–415–02846–9 (hbk)
ISBN 0–415–02847–7 (pbk)

Anorexic bodies

A feminist and sociological
perspective on anorexia nervosa

Morag MacSween

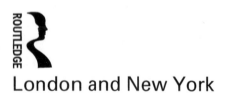

London and New York

Contents

Introduction

Twenty years ago very few people had heard of anorexia nervosa, an obscure psychiatric illness which seemed to confine itself almost exclusively to teenage girls. Since then anorexia has risen from its psychiatric obscurity to take its place in 'tabloidese'. Any woman who is well-known as well as thin has a reasonable chance of being diagnosed anorexic by journalistic pop psychologists. New theories about etiology and incidence – 'zinc cures' and anorexic yuppy men – are reported in the serious press. 'My triumph over anorexia' stories are common in women's magazines. Popular interest mirrors evidence of a real rise in cases of anorexia, with some estimates claiming that one in every hundred teenage girls is a sufferer. Many more are thought to develop the more covert disorder of bulimia, or teeter on the brink of anorexia.

For the sociologist and the feminist, too, anorexia is interesting. The anorexic 'boom' at precisely the time when feminism is again challenging the oppression of women, coupled with the evidence that almost all anorexics are women, that anorexia has a strong middle-class bias and that it is virtually unknown outside the developed West, suggest that the illness has some relationship to the social situation of middle-class women in modern Western culture. Most discussions of anorexia, whether psychiatric, feminist or popular, include at least some reference to the social position of women. Few, however, develop this suggested linkage into a fully sociological analysis of anorexia.

In trying to develop such an analysis, I want to avoid two common features of other writings on anorexia. The effects of the politics of physical appearance and the strictures of femininity on feminine psychology are frequent explanatory features in analyses of anorexia. However, with a few feminist exceptions this sociological perspective is simply 'added on' to explanations of anorexia as individual, or occasionally familial, pathology as though these two types of analysis were totally compatible. What is suggested is that while, yes, there are 'social pressures' on young women which impinge on their becoming anorexic, in the last instance it is a deficiency in the 'pre-anorexic' girl's psychology which explains anorexia. In this analysis, a sociological perspective on anorexia will be taken to its fullest extent.[1]

What I suggest, then, is that in the anorexic symptom women try to synthesize contradictory elements in their social position through the creation of an 'anorexic body'. In an early and influential feminist text Simone de Beauvoir argued:

> The terms *masculine* and *feminine* are used symmetrically only as a matter of form . . . In actuality the relation of the two sexes is not quite like that of two electrical poles, for man represents both the positive and the neutral, as is indicated by the common use of *man* to designate human beings in general; whereas woman represents only the negative . . . He is the Subject, he is the Absolute – she is the Other.
>
> (de Beauvoir, 1972: 15–16)

Maria Black and Rosalind Coward pick up on this point, arguing that:

> the attributes of the male can . . . disappear into a '*non-gendered*' subject. Women, on the other hand, never appear as non-gendered subjects. Women are precisely *defined*, never general representatives of human or all people, but as specifically feminine, and frequently sexual, categories: whore, slag, mother, virgin, housewife.
>
> (Black and Coward, 1981: 83)

Black and Coward point out, then, that definitions of femininity often centre on sexuality: women are 'the sex' (ibid.: 85). Women, further, are – in a significantly different way than men – bodies. De Beauvoir argues that social definitions of man as individual and woman as feminine resonate in our understandings of the body.[2] She suggests that the masculine body is thought to be 'a direct and normal connection with the world . . . apprehend(ed) objectively'; the feminine body, by contrast, is 'a hindrance, a prison, weighed down by everything peculiar to it' (de Beauvoir, 1972: 15). She quotes Benda: 'The body of man makes sense in itself quite apart from that of woman, whereas the latter seems wanting in significance by itself' (ibid.: 16).

Individuality is presented as gender-neutral but is fundamentally masculine. The social construction of gendered subjectivity conditions our perception of sexuality and of the body. My contention here is that just as 'individuality' and 'femininity' are understood by sociologists to be social constructions rather than naturally existing facts, so too are masculine and feminine desire and the masculine and feminine body. The self, the body and desire are socially constructed in the same structure of meaning: masculine is both masculine and neutral, and is active; feminine is only feminine, and is responsive.

The masculine/neutral self is constructed as independent: complete, separate and active. Masculine/neutral desire is constructed as active and possessive. The masculine/neutral body is constructed as impenetrable, active and intrusive; its imagery is of muscular action and phallic penetration. The feminine self is constructed as dependent: incomplete, responsive, seeking merger. Feminine desire is created as responsive; it allows possession but threatens to engulf. The feminine body is constructed as penetrable: simultaneously weak and threatening, its imagery is of orifices: mouth, vagina, womb.

As de Beauvoir points out, however, masculine and feminine are not polar opposites. Masculinity and femininity are defined interdependently, through a series of differences[3] or oppositions, but a third category – neutral – intervenes. In our equal opportunities culture a non-gendered subjectivity is – formally at least – 'available' for women, who are simultaneously non-gendered subjects and feminine objects. The superficial gender-neutrality of individuality masks its fundamentally masculine character. The social construction of masculine and feminine around *difference* means that being a man is 'not being a woman'; being a woman is 'not being a man'. Women who aspire to 'non-gendered' subjectivity undercut this structure of difference but rarely perceive it directly. Reconciling the hidden incompatibility between individuality and femininity is the central task of growing up female in contemporary Western culture.

It is this hidden incompatibility which lies, I would argue, at the heart of the anorexic symptom. The specific class and gender position of the 'anorexic population' addresses the dilemma of individuality and femininity particularly acutely. Her class position places expectations of educational and career success on the 'pre-anorexic' girl's shoulders (see Lawrence, 1984b). She must act in pursuit of her own interests. Her gender membership imprisons her within the constraints of femininity. She must respond to the needs and desires of others. The mutual exclusivity of these demands remains submerged in the ideology of gender-neutral individuality: their resolution, thus, is covert, subconscious, indirect.

Gender is created around three poles of difference: masculine, feminine and neutral. The social meanings of desire and the body are similarly constructed. In anorexia women take gender-neutral individuality seriously, working with the social constructions of feminine desire and the feminine body in an attempt to construct an *anorexic body* which resolves gender contradictions in being truly neutral.

This resolution commonly takes place at adolescence, a time of transition from childhood to adult life, the time when a personal assumption of an individual adult identity is required. Germaine Greer writes that 'the girl . . . struggles to reconcile her schooling along masculine lines with her feminine conditioning until puberty resolves the ambiguity and anchors her safely in the feminine posture, if it works' (Greer, 1971: 15). In the second era of public feminism the pressure to accept 'the feminine posture' faces severe challenges. Anorexia is one of the responses to this new situation which refuses to deny individuality in femininity.

The anorexic 'solution', however, is an indirect and individualized response to a *social* issue. Anorexic women cannot, in their isolation, produce a real or lasting solution to the degraded social construction of the feminine. As we shall see, their 'solution' is at best temporary and is always precarious. As one articulation of the irreconcilable social demands on women, the anorexic symptom, in spite of its ultimate strategic failure, does, however, offer a startling illumination of the lived realities of oppression.

In presenting a serious and detailed analysis of the anorexic symptom, therefore, I hope to further differentiate my analysis from those already on offer. As we shall see, both psychiatric and feminist explanations of anorexia tend to downgrade the actual anorexic process in analysis, focusing on the 'underlying' psychological dilemmas that are presumed to be expressed in anorexic behaviour rather than on the symptom itself. What this tends to imply is a rather arbitrary connection between the meaning and aims of anorexia and the activities through which those aims are expressed. Women's preoccupation with physical appearance in general and dieting in particular, plus their domestic responsibility for food explains why anorexic women choose food and the body as 'coping strategies'. 'Aim' and 'method' are thus relatively autonomous.

What I hope to show through a detailed analysis of *what anorexic women actually do* is that the meanings of anorexia are expressed *in*, rather than 'under' the symptom itself. It is no 'coincidence' that the anorexic conflict is expressed through the control of appetite and the attempt to create a needless and inviolate body, since the same structure of meaning constructs the body, the self and desire. The deconstruction of feminine appetite, then, is the central anorexic process: it is both aim and method.

My argument will be pursued in three parts. In Part I I look at existing analyses of anorexia, analysing the assumptions which underlie them as well as offering an outline of how anorexia is understood. Chapter 1 discusses the 'discovery' of anorexia by the nineteenth-century physicians Gull and Lasègue and traces the changes and continuities in dominant understandings of anorexia since it first became the object of psychiatric interest. In addition, this chapter criticizes the widely accepted assumption that anorexia has always existed, albeit in lesser 'quantities', pointing out, as do Cameron and Frazer in another context, that:

> We need to know not just what was done, but what it meant: the same act does not always have the same significance and to interpret the events of the past through the categories of the present is to make the error of historical anachronism.
>
> (Cameron and Frazer, 1987: 21)

Chapters 2 and 3 discuss, respectively, psychiatric and feminist explanations. Chapter 2 looks at the work of Arthur Crisp, Hilde Bruch, Roger Slade and Mara Selvini Palazzoli. There are, of course, significant theoretical divisions among these four writers. What they have in common is, however, the main focus of the chapter, which criticizes both 'individual pathology' explanations of anorexia and the recommendations for treatment which arise from it. In Chapter 3 I look at the work of Marilyn Lawrence, Susie Orbach and Kim Chernin, suggesting that while they significantly extend the analysis of anorexia in sociological terms, their work is undermined by a recognition of the contradictions of individuality and femininity which is only partial.

In Part II I outline the concepts through which anorexic women make sense of their experience, discussing my own interview material. This leads on to Part III, in which a feminist and fully sociological analysis of anorexia is outlined. Chapter 5 examines in detail the argument that the body should be seen as a social construction, relying heavily, though not uncritically, on Bryan Turner's introductory study. After a theoretical introduction I look at historical changes in the concept of the body, focusing on the effects of the gender division and the transition from feudalism to capitalism on dominant and oppositional body-concepts. Chapter 6 follows this up with a detailed analysis of contemporary understandings of the body, with specific reference to the construction of the feminine body through objectification and the control of feminine appetites. Chapter 7 suggests that the meanings and practices which were found to construct the feminine body are central to the anorexic experience, and demonstrates how.

A detailed analysis of the anorexic symptom is pursued through a discussion of anorexic women's responses to a questionnaire and the theoretical issues they raise. Here I argue that in anorexia women attempt a transformation of the degraded feminine body, disciplining their 'chaotic' appetites in the construction of a desireless anorexic body. The final chapter attempts to draw some preliminary conclusions on the social meaning of anorexia and what it tells us about the position of women in contemporary culture.

While I argue that historical changes in the mode of production and class divisions are vital elements in a sociological analysis of anorexia, I do see anorexia as fundamentally about gender. The social construction of the gender division thus takes centre stage in my analysis, and I make use of the contested concept of patriarchy (see e.g. Beechey, 1979; Rowbotham, 1979; Alexander and Taylor, 1980; Barrett, 1980; Segal, 1987). The concept of patriarchy has been criticized as suggesting that the oppression of women is monolithic and unchanging. This is not my intention in using the concept, and I explicitly argue that the construction of femininity and the social control of women vary with historical change, class divisions and racist categorizations. I use patriarchy, then, to signify the continuing oppression of women as a gender through changes in the mode of production and across divisions of class and ethnic background, rather than as a means of ignoring their existence. As Black and Coward argue:

> The women's movement takes its existence from the fact that however differently we are constituted in different practices and discourses, women are constantly and inescapably constructed *as women*.
>
> (Black and Coward, 1981: 85)

In Chapter 5 I argue that the social construction of 'woman' underwent a transformation with the transition from feudalism to capitalism. This definitional change took place, however, through a framework of continuity which constructs women, and specifically women's sexuality, as a threat to male order, however that order is constituted. Female 'formlessness' is differentiated from male order, as Genevieve Lloyd argues, tracing the Western philosophical association of women with nature and male with culture, the 'longstanding associations between maleness and form, femaleness and matter' (Lloyd, 1984: 5). In discussing the body, the patriarchal definition of woman as structureless matter is central. Mary Ellmann argues that:

> The impression of woman's formlessness underlies the familiar . . . acknowledgment of their superficial form. It is of course a physiological impression, and the sexual analogy is transparent: soft body, soft mind. The flesh of woman (as Sade would put it) is less resistant and less muscular than that of man. Pinched, it bruises more easily. And if it is impressionable, the impressionable mind must be not only beyond pinching but beyond form. It cannot maintain even so lax a hold upon itself as the body does. There, in the mind, all is liquid and drowning. Solid ground is masculine, the sea is feminine.
>
> (Ellmann, 1979: 74)

It is one aim of the subsequent discussion to trace the continuity of the notion of formlessness of woman through changing concepts of the body, arguing that patriarchal constructions of the feminine body, in opposing feminine matter to masculine form, understand the feminine body as weak and penetrable but simultaneously as potentially powerful and engulfing. A social constructionist approach to the body would argue, against Ellmann, that the body can be equally as 'liquid and drowning' as the mind. It is the construction of the feminine body as limitless – a patriarchal construction – with which the anorexic symptom engages.

Since my argument is that in anorexia women transform the social meanings and practices through which the feminine body is constructed, a detailed analysis of anorexic meanings and practices must be central. Although the argument is pursued in the main theoretically, the two chapters which examine anorexic practices and the concepts through which anorexic women make sense of their experience rely on my own interviews with anorexic women and on replies to a questionnaire.[4]

I interviewed eight anorexic women and one bulimic woman, and this material forms the basis of Chapter 4. Here my intention is to uncover anorexic meanings, and I present the interview material in a modified case-study format. One case study is discussed in depth, and the central concepts which emerge from it are followed up in the words of five other women. Here feelings of control, powerlessness, pride, guilt, pressure and shame emerge as central.

In addition I used a postal questionnaire in order to discover the exact mechanisms of anorexia. This proved to be an excellent way to find out in detail what anorexic women actually do. Obviously talking about issues like the kind of food women eat and don't eat, how they plan their eating, and what binges involve is extremely difficult for anorexic women, and the anonymity of the questionnaire form allowed many of the respondents to be remarkably frank. This material is analysed in Chapter 7. In both chapters women's names have been changed.

Approximately half of the women I interviewed had attended Anorexic Aid self-help groups. The others either replied to the questionnaire and lived near enough to be interviewed or were introduced by other interviewees. The women who replied to the questionnaire responded to an advert in the Anorexic Aid magazine; 38 women replied to the advert and in the end 35 completed questionnaires. Obviously this material in no way allows me to draw generalized conclusions about anorexia: the sample is non-random and fairly small. So this material is not intended to 'prove' a hypothesis, but is used to explore and exemplify a theoretical argument. As Elizabeth Frazer points out, with small samples – and, in this case, with non-random ones – '"findings" have to be seen as suggestive rather than demonstrative; and quantitative analysis is quite inappropriate' (Frazer, 1988: 345). Further, as Mica Satow points out:

> whatever data you are working with it is actually going to be subject to your own translation . . . as researchers we bring to the material that we are going to translate not only our own personal histories but also a very real politics. Nothing is neutral once we have put our hands on it and once we have put our minds to it.
>
> (Satow, 1987: 8)

The words and writing of the women I quote appear, therefore, as translations rather than direct 'realities'. I chose which questions to ask and I edited the answers; the perspective which their ideas support is mine not theirs. From talking to the women I interviewed and reading their responses to the questionnaire I am aware that their individual understandings of anorexia differ, in greater or lesser degrees, from mine. I hope they will feel that their ideas have been treated with respect, especially in cases where the theoretical and political gulf between their perspective and mine was greatest.

Part I

Explaining anorexia

Chapter 1

Anorexia nervosa
The history of the concept

The term 'anorexia nervosa' was coined in 1873 by an English physician, William Gull. In an 'aside' in the Address in Medicine to the British Medical Association in 1868 he had referred to some cases of emaciation occurring without evident organic cause in young women, terming this 'apepsia hysterica' (digestive problems of hysterical origin) (Gull, 1868: 175). Five years later he changed the term to 'anorexia nervosa', the latter term 'more fairly expressing the facts, since what food is taken, except in the extreme stages of the disease, is well digested' (Gull, 1873: 534).

It is worth quoting Gull's original description of anorexia at some length as, apart from the obvious terminological updating, this description contains most of the essential characteristics of anorexia recognized by contemporary psychiatry.

In anorexia, for Gull, 'the want of appetite is due to a morbid mental state', a 'want of mental equilibrium', occurring in a group – young women between 15 and 23 – who were well known to be 'specially obnoxious to mental perversity' (ibid.: 535; 1874: 25). No signs of organic disease were evident either during the illness or in post-mortems. The patients complained neither of pain nor hunger, and were often 'restless and wayward'. This, argued Gull, 'was . . . a striking expression of the nervous state, for it seemed hardly possible that a body so wasted could undergo the exercise which seemed agreeable' (Gull, 1874: 23).

The treatment Gull advocated was 'moral control', through which the patient's 'mental equilibrium' was to be brought back into balance (Gull, 1873: 534–5). 'Medical' treatment as such did not contribute much to recovery, but a strict feeding programme, which paid no heed to the desires of the patient, was to be adhered to (Gull, 1874: 24). Gull explains the necessity for 'moral' treat-ment:

> I have remarked ... that these wilful patients are often allowed
> to drift their own way into a state of extreme exhaustion, when
> it might have been prevented by placing them under different
> moral conditions. The treatment required is obviously that
> which is fitted for persons of unsound mind. The patients
> should be fed at regular intervals, and surrounded by persons
> who would have moral control over them; relations and friends
> being generally the worst attendants.
>
> (ibid.: 26)

In advocating 'moral' treatment, Gull was not suggesting any new
or dramatic treatment for anorexic women. The idea that the mad
could be cured rather than simply confined had arisen in the
second half of the eighteenth century and in the next century cure
essentially came to mean 'moral management'. Here, the complete
control of the patient's behaviour and environment by the physician was intended to lead to the development of self-restraint and
a return to mental equilibrium, with lack of restraint and 'extreme'
habits and behaviour being held to be central in the development
of madness (Foucault, 1965; Skultans, 1979; Doerner, 1981; Scull,
1981). Foucault and Doerner both argue that the family was used
as a 'moral model' in this treatment. Doerner argues that 'the
insane asylum ... retained the aura of a simulated family' (1981:
81), and Foucault suggests that within asylums 'the social structure
of the bourgeois family' was reconstructed (1965: 257). The doctor
and the asylum were to accomplish what the father and the home
had failed to achieve – the internalization of bourgeois social
morality (ibid.: 257–60).

Asked at the Clinical Society whether the line between anorexia
and 'real insanity' was difficult to establish, Gull replied that 'there
was perhaps no great amount of hysteria, but it could hardly be
called insanity' (Gull, 1873: 535).

At more or less the same time, and independently of William
Gull, the French phsyician Ernest Lasègue introduced the disease
'hysterical anorexia' to the medical establishment. Lasègue sought
to differentiate anorexia from the large category of hysterical
disorders, proceeding through this 'somewhat diagrammatic
sketch':

A young girl, between 15 and 20 years of age, suffers from some emotion which she avows or conceals. Generally it relates to some real or imaginary marriage proposal, to a violence done to some sympathy, or to some more or less conscious desire . . . at first, she feels uneasiness after food, vague sensations of fullness, suffering and gastralgia post-prandium, or rather coming on from the commencement of the repast . . . the patient thinks to herself that the best remedy for this indefinite and painful uneasiness will be to diminish her food. Up to this point there is nothing remarkable in her case, for almost every sufferer from gastralgia has submitted to this temptation . . . With the hysterical things take another course. Gradually she reduces her food, furnishing pretexts . . . at the end of some weeks there is no longer a supposed temporary repugnance, but a refusal of food that may be indefinitely prolonged.

(Lasègue, 1873: 265)

This course is then pursued 'with implacable tenacity', the patient claiming that she is neither ill nor thinner (ibid.: 265).

The central features of anorexia, for Gull and Lasègue, as for contemporary psychiatry, are, then: emaciation, occurring without organic causation; a specific distribution, by age and by gender (although the *class* distribution was not noticed by Gull and Lasègue); the denial by the patient that she was ill, and the corresponding recognition of a degree of conscious *choice* in anorexia; and a view of anorexia as a non-organic disorder. In treatment too, there are broad similarities – refeeding and 'moral' treatment under the direction of medical professionals in the nineteenth century, and refeeding plus psychotherapy for modern psychiatry – both courses in which medical control of the environment and behaviour of the patient is the object.

However, one major difference should be noted. Gull, as we have seen, suggested that the anorexic girl had no appetite for food, and Lasègue argued that a positive *aversion* to food existed. The contemporary concensus is that 'anorexia' – lack of appetite – is a misnomer, as the anorexic woman *does* still experience hunger, and her appetite remains 'normal'.

After the initial articles by Gull and Lasègue appeared, while some comments and additions were made – including those of Charcot, Huchard and Janet (Palazzoli, 1974: 6) – the accepted and unquestioned definition of anorexia (still very much a rare 'minority' disease) was theirs. As Palazzoli argues:

> By the turn of the century it was widely agreed that anorexia was a mental illness. In particular most authorities believed that the patients' obstinate refusal to take food under all sorts of pretexts and the resulting inanition, were the sole causes of the severe and often fatal organic sequelae of the disease.
>
> (ibid.: 7)

This view remained dominant until 1914 when Morris Simmonds described a case of death from starvation in which the pituitary was found to be damaged. This led to a labelling of the still infrequent cases of anorexia as 'Simmonds' Disease', and the term anorexia and the acceptance of psychological causation all but disappeared. It was not until the late 1930s that the distinction between Simmonds' Disease – starvation due to pituitary malfunction – and anorexia – starvation deliberately chosen – was redrawn (ibid.: 7–8). And it was not until the publication of the study by Sheehan and Summers in 1949 which showed that pituitary gland atrophy and hypothalamic symptoms were not causally related that the controversy finally ended (see Morgan, 1977).

Up until the 1960s, however, anorexia was still viewed as a relatively rare condition, and it is really in the last thirty years that the vast increase of interest in and work on anorexia has occurred. Hilde Bruch, for example, refers to anorexia as a 'new' disease because of what she argues is a rapidly increasing incidence since 1960, an incidence which she relates to media pressures on young women to slim (Bruch, 1978: vii–viii).

In my own analysis I shall also treat anorexia as a 'twentieth-century' phenomenon, but for somewhat more complex reasons, as the introduction has suggested. I shall argue that the social context in which anorexia can arise as a meaningful existential strategy, while originating in the late nineteenth century with the first 'modern' wave of female aspiration to patriarchal individualism (in, especially, the demands for education and political rights for women), has only in the post-war period intensified and widened its social base to the extent that the contradictory pressures of 'femininity' and 'success' are felt by the majority of young middle-class girls.

IS THE HISTORY OF THE CONCEPT THE HISTORY OF THE DISEASE?

Part of the proliferation of research into anorexia has been an attempt to establish the existence of cases before 1873 by 're-diagnosing' cases of voluntary starvation in young women as anorexia. This strategy can be seen to follow from the idea of a fixed and unchanging 'human nature', the dilemmas of which are seen as universal. As Ritenbaugh argues:

> the fact that biomedicine does not include culture in its basic explanatory model leads to . . . a redefinition of syndromes from other cultures into biomedical terms so that potentially important cultural patterns [may] become irrelevant to diagnosis or treatment.
>
> (Quoted in Swartz, 1985: 34)

Specifically on anorexia, the current psychiatric view is that anorexia has always existed, but has only recently been 'discovered', due to increased medical knowledge and/or increased prevalence. Bruch, as we have seen, points to media pressures on young women to slim, and Crisp (1974) argues that better nutrition leading to earlier puberty combined with twentieth-century moral uncertainty can lead to anorexia. Slade (1984), Crisp (1974) and Wellbourne and Purgold (1984) all argue that anorexia has in all likelihood always existed, and Sheila Macleod (1981: 13) finds it hard to believe that there have not always been 'emotionally isolated young girls like myself pursuing the same lonely course'.

This view, and the arguments that back it up, are founded not only on an essentialist but also on a *behaviourist* understanding of human psychology. All that seems to be necessary in this 're-diagnosis' is the presence of starvation without evident organic cause. The *meanings* of that starvation, and the possibility that such meanings refer to and change with specific social contexts are conspicuous by their absence.

I would argue that two misconceptions are operating here. First, this view is ahistorical. Second, the distinction between *action* and *meaning* is crucially blurred. Human behaviour and personality are assumed to be more or less constant over time, the atomized individualism of bourgeois society being naturalized as eternally existing 'human nature', and seen as inherent, rather than created in social relations. Further, it is assumed that all non-organically based starvation, especially if voluntarily under-taken, *is* anorexia. I would argue, against this view, that the *meanings* entailed in the control of food and the body can and do change, both historically and gender-specifically.

Thus, arguing that anorexia nervosa as a reaction to the prob-lems of adolescence for girls is a universal phenomenon is untenable. 'Adolescence' is itself a historically specific category, as Philippe Ariès has shown (Ariès, 1973); the 'adolescent crisis' is a specifically twentieth-century problem, and is, as shall later be argued, dependent on a specific social construction of individ-uality.

To develop and ground the argument above, I would like to go on to look in depth at the 'pre-concept' case most often said to be anorexia,[1] and then to consider Bell's argument that anorexia was a striking feature of the medieval female religious experience (Bell, 1985).

Anorexia in the seventeenth century? Richard Morton's *Pthisiologia*

Pthisiologia: Or, a Treatise of Consumptions, written by Richard Mor-ton, a fellow of the College of Physicians, was published in 1694. In this work, Morton distinguished somatic and psychological consumptions. 'Nervous' consumption was due, he argued, to 'an ill and morbid state of the Spirits', a weakness or destruction of 'the Tone of the Nerves', the fever, coughing and shortness of breath of ordinary consumption being absent:

> In the beginning of this Disease the state of the Body appears oedematous and blouted and as if it were stuffed with dispirited Chyle; the face is pale and squalid, the Stomack loathes every-thing but Liquids.
>
> (Morton, 1694: 2–4)

The lack of appetite and bad digestion occur because the 'morbid state' of the nerves hinders the 'Assimilation, Fermentation and Volatilization' of gastric juices. This state of the nerves can be accounted for by 'violent Passions of the Mind', drinking and bad air (ibid.: 5). The patient should: 'endeavour to divert and make his mind cheerful by Exercise, and the Conversation of his Friends. For this Disease does almost always preceed from Sadness, and anxious cares' (ibid.: 7). Also, various 'stomach medicines' could be prescribed (ibid.: 6).

Morton details two case histories, the first of which forms the basis for the claim that 'nervous consumption' was in fact anorexia nervosa. He writes:

> Mr. Duke's Daughter in St. Mary Axe, in the year 1694, and in the Eighteenth Year of her Age, in the Month of July fell into a total suppression of her Monthly Courses from a Multitude of Care and Passions of her Mind, but without any symptom of the Green Sickness following upon it. From which time her Appetite began to abate, and her Digestion to be bad . . . she was wont by her studying at Night, and continual poring upon Books, to expose herself both Day and Night to the injuries of the Air, which was at that time extremely cold . . . I do not remember that I did ever in all my Practice see one, that was conversant with the Living so much wasted with the greatest degree of a Consumption . . . like a skeleton only clad with skin.
> (ibid.: 8–9)

Morton did not view 'nervous consumption' as a specifically female disease. Indeed, in its association with sadness and studiousness, nervous consumption would have been more likely to have been associated with the *male* disease of melancholy by Morton and his contemporaries.

I would suggest that it is at the very least tenuous to describe this case as anorexia. There is very little actual evidence on which to base such an assumption; we are in no position to assume that the lack of appetite which Morton saw as central did not in fact exist. Even if one were to accept the logic of historically constant illness categories, unaffected by culture, there is nothing in Morton to distinguish his case as anorexia rather than one of the other psychiatric conditions in which lack of appetite or delusions about food feature (see Morgan, 1977: 1652).

Fundamentally, however, the central feature of anorexia – the deliberate and conscious maintenance of food control – is not mentioned in Morton's case history. It should not be 'forced in' in retrospect, and without it, the case for re-diagnosing 'Mr Duke's daughter' as an early anorexic does not hold water.

Anorexia in the fourteenth century? Bell's *Holy Anorexia*

In a review of *Holy Anorexia* in the *Observer*, Lorna Sage (1986) tells us that Bell 'has looked into the lives of Italian female saints, blesseds and venerables, to find evidence that they had this supposedly faddy modern disease'. Bell himself is more cautious, arguing for a distinction between anorexia nervosa and 'holy anorexia'. He argues:

> the modifier is the key; whether anorexia is holy or nervous depends on the culture in which a young woman strives to gain control of her life. In both cases anorexia begins as the girl fastens onto a highly valued societal goal – bodily health/thinness/self-control in the twentieth century, spiritual health, self-denial and fasting in medieval Christendom . . . Insecurity (I am no one/I am a worthless, debased sinner) gives way to absolute certainty . . . each pursues her externally different but psychologically analogous, culturally approved objective with fanatical, compulsive devotion.
>
> (Bell, 1985: 20–1)

Looked at more closely, then, the distinction between anorexias nervosa and holy is one of *style* rather than *substance*. Bell sees anorexia as arising from an 'adolescent crisis', in which the young girl seeks an autonomy of action which her culture proscribes (ibid.: 40). The struggle for true autonomy in the outside world being unwinnable, the anorexic internalizes the struggle into one with her own body. Although it is disguised as a struggle to achieve a socially valued goal – holiness for the medieval, thinness for the modern anorexic – the *real* struggle is for autonomy, self-sufficiency and a sense of self, and 'in this sense the anorexic response is timeless' (ibid.: 56). It is, then, in the intersection of this static and universal psychological need with changing 'cultural imperatives' that the differing forms or styles of anorexia are created (ibid.: 21).

Bell identifies numerous cases, from the twelfth to the seventeenth centuries, of Italian nuns starving themselves, sometimes to death, but in any case to a degree far beyond the fasting recognized by the Church, and he argues that it was in the fourteenth century that this 'holy anorexia' reached its peak. Of these women, the best known, and the one which Bell treats in most depth is Catherine Benincasa, later St Catherine of Siena.

Her fasting, he argues, was renowned, became a model for others through the publication of her *Life*, and was something of a thorn in the flesh of her confessors and the Church authorities, as Catherine frequently claimed that she could not moderate her behaviour, even when told it was vainglorious not to. When ordered to eat, she did, but she vomited if even a mouthful of food remained in her stomach, and for long periods she was reputed to eat nothing at all. It is from this evidence, then, that Bell treats Catherine as his paradigmatic medieval anorexic (ibid.: 23–7).

He suggests that Catherine's anorexia had domestic causes. Catherine was born a twin, and her sickly sister Giovanna was sent out to a wet nurse, while she herself was fed by their mother. The twin soon died, while Catherine, the favoured child, flourished. Further, when Catherine was 15, her older sister Bonaventura died in childbirth. Bell surmises that guilt at the first death, and the realization at the second of the possible consequences of a dutiful secular female life led Catherine to abandon the world and take to 'radical holiness', both as an alternative to marriage and as a penance to ensure that no more of her family would suffer an early death (ibid.: 29–46).

After a struggle against her family's marriage plans, Catherine joined the Sisters of Penance, a Dominican Order of women who lived at home 'in the world' rather than in a convent, and she dedicated herself to the religious life. Her ascetic practices continued and intensified once she had achieved her goal of the religious life. She continually limited her food, often eating only bread and water and sometimes fasting totally. However, it is clear from Bell's own description that starvation, far from being a goal in itself, was, for Catherine, merely one part of a life of asceticism. As Bell himself points out, *all* bodily urges were for Catherine 'base obstructions in her path of holiness' (ibid.: 15). He persists in focusing on her attitudes to food, glossing over her other mortifications of the flesh – wearing an iron chain round her hips which cuts into her flesh, self-flagellation, drinking pus, and walking with thirty-three small stones in her shoes (ibid.: 19, 25, 43–4).

This narrow concentration on Catherine's eating habits, I would argue, shows Bell's desire to force her asceticism to fit anorexic symptomatology. Why else should not eating be picked out of the catalogue of Catherine's physical self-torments? Similarly, and amazingly for a religious historian, he all but disregards the *religious* rationale for asceticism, arguing that: 'Notwithstanding the vast differences between Catherine's desire to be united with God and the modern day anorexic's quest for a sense of self, the psychological dilemma is similar' (ibid.: 28).

Bell explains Catherine's dilemma as having familial and psychological causes – as, he argues, does anorexia nervosa. The assumption here is that the path from childhood via adolescence to adulthood is determined by an innate psychology whose effects far outweigh mere historical contingencies like belief in the supernatural. However, as I mentioned above, this is far from being the case. Ariès, for example, in his influential *Centuries of Childhood*, effectively demonstrates that *social* childhood, as distinct from biological development, is a culturally constructed entity whose characteristics vary with and are defined by the wider social structure (Ariès, 1973). The category 'adolescence' is a relatively recent one, and depends on the existence of an identifiable intermediate period between the complete dependency of childhood and the independence of adulthood. To argue, as Bell does, that the 'adolescent' struggle to define the self as independent of the family unit is an essential feature of human development is, then, both ahistorical and misconceived.

Further, Bell manages to almost ignore the deep and all-encompassing effects of religious belief in the medieval period. As Southern (1970: 16) points out, the medieval church was 'a compulsory society'. Bell argues, for example, that Catherine chose to join a tertiary order in order that she could remain with her family – 'the only context that meant anything to her' (Bell, 1985: 48). Does this suggest that her desire for union with God is not to be taken seriously?

Bell seems to suggest that only those who *themselves* believe in the supernatural could give credence to a supernatural motivation for Catherine's asceticism – her expressed desire to transcend the world and the flesh and be united with Christ (ibid.: 29). The implicit argument seems to be that the *real* dilemmas of humanity are those of individualism, and that although the medieval ascetic believed herself to be seeking union with God, this was in reality a cloak to her *true* desire for 'individual autonomy'.

I would argue, against Bell, that it requires not a belief in the supernatural, but a respect for history to 'take seriously' the religious motivations of Catherine and the other 'holy anorexics'. They did not create the system of meanings within which the body was deemed corrupt and trancendence a reality – rather, these were the *social* meanings of the medieval period, meanings in which ascetic practices of all kinds were framed.[2] As Bell himself points out of Catherine: 'in the spiritual world her accomplishments are magnificent. She becomes Christ's bride . . . and regularly communicates with Him, with Mary and with the Heavenly Host' (ibid.: 20). One does not have to accept that this 'really happened' in order to accept it as her *real* motivation in the attempt to transcend the body. As Bolton writes of medieval 'holy virgins': 'their physical detachment opens up an immense capacity for loving their Lord and the renunciation of temporal goods reveals an unassuaged desire for real and eternal goods' (Bolton, 1978: 266).

In short, then, I would argue that Bell's project is fundamentally misconceived. He abstracts from an entire system of ascetic practices one which can be forced into analogy with what is essentially a modern disease category, and explains it without regard to the context in which it arose – the 'well-marked . . . path of saintly austerity . . . [whose] . . . rewards are ultimate' (Bell, 1985: 13). It was the *world*, not just food, which Catherine rejected. Bell's argument relies on the acceptance of a universal psychological development process, and is thus ahistorical. Although there *are* interesting parallels between religious asceticism in the medieval period and anorexia as a modern asceticism, and although patriarchal constraint is central for both the medieval religious ascetic and the modern anorexic, anorexia and 'holy anorexia' are not the same thing.

For the modern anorexic, the path is lonely and the reward questionable. She does not have the social 'back-up' which Catherine of Siena had, and the 'self' which is meaningful to her would be an alien concept to a medieval nun. The self is not a historical constant which 'intersects' with an external culture, but rather itself derives its meaning from and is shaped by that culture. This is what Bell forgets, assuming as he does that the unique and self-contained self has always been the proper quest of humanity.

Chapter 2

The enigma variations
Psychiatric explanations of anorexia

INTRODUCTION

In her article 'Current approaches to the etiology and treatment of anorexia nervosa', Kelly M. Bemis outlines four main psychiatric approaches to anorexia: psychodynamic, family interactional, behavioural and medical. The psychodynamic approach sees anorexia as a disorder of the individual psyche, in which the refusal of food is symbolic of some other, deeper fear or anxiety. The family interactional approach sees anorexia as a power-strategy within a system of family relations, concentrating on the perceived function, rather than the content of anorexic behaviour. The behavioural approach sees anorexia as a learned response which can be 'unlearned', discarding any attempt to analyse the meaning or dynamics of anorexia. Finally, the medical model concentrates on the somatic elements of anorexia, research aiming at the discovery of an underlying physiological cause (Bemis, 1978).

As outlined in the introduction, my own work will concentrate on an attempt to render anorexia nervosa explicable, to uncover how the dominant social conceptualizations of food and the body are transformed in anorexia. From this perspective, therefore, my review of the psychiatric definitions of anorexia will concentrate on the psychodynamic approach, with some coverage of the medical approach, as this is the strand in psychiatry which treats *explanation* of anorexia most centrally, the family interactional approach looking at function rather than meaning, and the behavioural approach disregarding entirely the search for understanding, concentrating as it does on 'cure' through reward and punishment. I have chosen to look at the medical approach *not* out of an acceptance of theories of organic causation but because consideration of the ways in which the somatic components of anorexia are given meaning will be central to my own analysis.

With this in mind, therefore, I will focus on the work of four psychiatrists – Hilde Bruch, A.H. Crisp, Roger Slade and Mara Selvini Palazzoli. Bruch and Crisp are leading authorities on anorexia in, respectively, the US and Britain, and have been working and writing on anorexia since the early 1960s. Bruch's work is almost entirely psychodynamic, in that she sees stringent food control as an attempt to impose in one area the personal control that the anorexic girl feels she lacks in her life as a whole. Crisp's work straddles the medical and psychodynamic approaches, explaining anorexia as a retreat into childhood from both the physical and social/psychological consequences of adolescence. Palazzoli, an Italian psychologist, has recently moved into the area of family therapy, but it is her earlier analysis of anorexia which I wish to look at, focusing as it does on the bodily experience of the anorexic woman. Lastly, I have chosen to look at the work of Roger Slade because it contains an intriguing attempt to synthesize notions of both organic and psychological causation.

After outlining the main features of each of these explanations of anorexia, I shall go on to criticize them from a sociological and feminist perspective, unearthing the hidden assumptions about 'sanity' and 'normality' which inform them – in Smith's terms, 'the invisible judgemental work' of psychiatric theorizing (quoted in Penfold and Walker, 1983: 42). I will argue that 'scientific' psychiatric analyses contain an unquestioned and unanalysed set of 'common-sense' assumptions about 'normality' – that, in short, being 'normal' or 'sane' means being able to function appropriately in a bourgeois patriarchal culture. Here, 'normality' is taken to be a naturally existing fact, rather than a socially constructed concept (ibid.: 39).

The dominant definition of mental illness in bourgeois culture is of a purely *personal* and *internal* phenomenon, resulting either from biochemical irregularities or internal psychological 'maladjustment'. The mentally ill person cannot adjust to the normal world – for a variety of reasons – and so must be institutionalized and 'readjusted' – in a variety of ways. Failure to adjust is seen as a problem of *individual* deviance, as what we must adjust *to* is unquestioned, and seen, therefore, as natural, attainable and essentially unproblematic except for the deviant minority.

However, acceptable 'normal' behaviour is by no means a

gender-neutral standard. Phyllis Chesler cites the Broverman studies to illustrate this point (Broverman, 1970, 1972; Chesler, 1974). In these studies, a questionnaire was given to psychiatric clinicians which consisted of a list of behaviours and character traits which the clinicians were to apply to the standards of 'healthy male', 'healthy female' and 'healthy adult' behaviour. Chesler points out:

> [their] concepts of healthy mature men did not differ significantly from their concepts of healthy mature adults, but their concepts of healthy mature women did differ significantly from those for men and for adults . . . [W]omen differ . . . by being more submissive, less independent, less adventurous, more easily influenced, less aggressive, less competitive, more excitable about minor crises, more easily hurt, more emotional, more conceited about their appearances, less objective and less interested in maths and science.

(Chesler, 1974: 65)

The implications of this for women are that to be seen as mentally healthy women must adjust to a standard of behaviour that is held to be acceptable for women but not desirable either for men or for adults. Chesler argues from this that 'the ethic of mental health is masculine in our culture' and that 'only men can be mentally healthy' (ibid.: 65, 64). However, that the standards of *adult* mental health are 'adapted' for women does *not* mean that women are 'immune' to the expectations of the unadapted adult/masculine standard. Women are, in effect, caught in a double-bind of having to fit in with *both* sets of expectations – to be an independent, self-contained individual as well as being feminine, and thus organizing their activities mainly towards the needs of others. For women, there is 'a double standard of mental health' (ibid.: xix).

There is, I would argue, a constant tension between the bourgeois idea of the atomized and self-subsistent individual (an idea developed in the context of patriarchy) and the specific patriarchal demands on women, expressed in the concept of 'femininity'. This tension is one which psychiatry, in viewing as 'natural' and eternal the gender roles and personality structures of bourgeois patriarchy, cannot fully 'see'.[1]

In my discussions of the psychiatric explanations of anorexia, then, I will be focusing on the underlying assumption that 'normality' is achievable – that the personal assumption of the conflicting demands of being both adult and female at adolescence is a process that only the ill or deviant individual will find seriously problematic – and the effect of this on subsequent theorizing. As Penfold and Walker write: 'once a person is suspected or diagnosed as mentally ill, she becomes someone who is not expected to make sense in terms of the social definition of rationality or normality' (Penfold and Walker: 1983, 42).

Psychiatric explanations of anorexia thus start from the premise that anorexia as a behaviour will not 'make sense' in any profound way, and this severely limits the extent to which any real understanding can be developed. Indeed, as we shall see, analysis of the anorexic *symptom* itself takes a definite second place behind analysis of the psychological dilemmas and inadequacies which are presumed to underlie it. These underlying issues, I will argue, are constructed through a taken-for-granted concept of individuality and individual development which is ahistorical and phallocentric.

ARTHUR CRISP: ANOREXIA AS BIOLOGICAL REGRESSION

Anorexia, for Crisp, is 'a phobic avoidance stance', 'a distorted biological solution to an existential problem for an adolescent' (Crisp, 1980: preface, 91).

The phobia for the anorexic is of *herself* at normal (average) adolescent body-weight. Her often expressed fear of 'fatness' hides the change in meaning of the word 'fat' for the anorexic, to whom 'fat' equals normal adolescent bodyweight (Crisp and Fransella, 1972: 395; Crisp, 1967: 716; 1970b: 493). The anorexic state represents a 'psychobiological regression', a 'flight back into psychobiological childhood', and is, as such, an *adaptive* state which protects the individual in whom puberty and its attendant 'maturational crisis' have been experienced as overwhelming (Crisp, 1974: 530; 1970b: 454; 1979: 149, 63). It is thus the control of *weight* and *shape*, not of eating or food, that is central, the aim being to regain and maintain a sub-pubertal body-weight. Crisp argues that anorexic women, if they could eat without gaining weight, would do so, as the only significance of food in anorexia arises from its relationship to weight and shape (Crisp *et al.*, 1977: 63; Crisp, 1980: 14–15, 78).

The anorexic girl, then, regresses into psychobiological childhood in order to avoid the 'existential challenge' of puberty (1980:

48). It is puberty that introduces weight and shape as meaningful and threatening, as it is the crossing of a relatively precise weight threshold which causes the 'qualitative biological and psychosocial changes' of puberty to occur (1980: 78). Of central significance are the development of secondary sexual characteristics – in girls, the development of breasts, pubic hair, the laying down of fat on buttocks, stomach, thighs and upper arms, and the menarche – which result from increased production of 'sex' hormones. This 'normal' female 'fatness' is profoundly significant both biologically and socially; biologically in that it signals that the girl is reproductively capable, and socially in that it arouses male sexual interest (1980: 38; 1979: 150).

Concomitant to sexual development is an adolescent appetite surge, which provides the necessary energy and growth to push the adolescent over this threshold weight at which the biological mechanisms in the brain governing sex-hormone activity are 'switched on' (1980: 84). Thus, Crisp argues, 'eating becomes particularly equated with emerging sexuality through its symbolic link . . . [and] . . . its biological primacy over the latter [sexuality]' (1980: 46). Food control is, therefore, the obvious course for the adolescent who seeks a retreat from maturation.

What, then, is the precise nature of this 'maturational crisis'; and what is specific in it for girls in general and 'pre-anorexic' girls in particular?

For Crisp, as we have seen, puberty is primarily a physiological event, with a secondary and dependent 'social' element. Sexuality, for Crisp, emerges at adolescence as a result of the increase in hormonal production; sexual feelings and urges are a *biological* creation. 'Adolescent turmoil' is 'an inevitable accompaniment of the processes of post-pubertal growth' (1974: 532). Puberty, then, as a primarily physiological event, 'intrudes massively into the world of the child and demands that the sense of self enlarge so as to incorporate sexuality and decay' (1980: 49). The adolescent must forge a sense of self which includes the integration and control of sexual and other impulses, independence from parents and a secure sense of his/her feelings and needs (Crisp and Fransella, 1972: 395; Crisp, 1983b). This is a time of change and experimentation, the successful resolution of which results in 'a well-developed sense of the self' (1980: 58).

The 'social' element in puberty/adolescence is twofold. First, the adolescent self must be developed 'in ways adaptive to the available social matrix' (1980: 49). Second, today's adolescent is faced, Crisp argues, with a permissive society in which guidelines for behaviour and social rules are lacking, in which there is 'philosophical and moral uncertainty and bankruptcy' (1974: 530; see also 1979: 150; 1980: 60–1; 1981–2: 213). Thus, there is a need for greater structure and stronger controls *within* the self (1983a: 857; 1980: 60), and while this is positive for most, for the few it is problematic: insecurity in values 'may allow the more robust amongst us to develop to the maximum . . . [but] . . . for the more vulnerable it is probably very difficult indeed' (1979: 150).

Thus far, then, the maturational crisis applies to all 'modern' adolescents,[2] is unavoidable and, it is implied, is usually successfully negotiated.

For girls, however, there are extra problems. As well as the more complex hormonal and physiological processes involved in female pubertal development, there are specific psychosexual problems for the female adolescent. Unfortunately, Crisp assumes that these problems are so well known to the reader that he does not list or explain them, except for a brief mention of the risk of pregnancy (1968: 370). Neither does he expand on the 'different, and often less immediately challenging psychosexual implications of adolescence for the male' (1970b: 466). It is, however, safe to assume that, for Crisp, sexuality is seen simply as more of a problem for girls, the word 'overwhelming' cropping up fairly regularly (i.e. 1970b: 494–5). It is these special problems, coupled with the very strong preoccupation among teenage girls with weight, shape and attractiveness, which make the anorexic retreat from maturity – in which the central motive is, in Eardner's words, 'to stalemate physiological growth in the sexual sphere' – a more 'female' course, adolescent turmoil becoming construed solely in terms of body shape (1970b: 454; 1980: 24–5, 142; Crisp *et al.*, 1980: 230).

So, having accounted for the specificity of the adolescent maturational crisis for girls in general, how does Crisp then account for the differential experience of the crisis in non-anorexic and pre-anorexic girls? His explanation is twofold. First, anorexics' families can be pathological in a variety of ways; and second, it can be the anorexic herself who is deficient in some way: anorexia can be caused either by the two acting together, or by the second alone (Crisp *et al.*, 1977: 66).

First, then, in some families the crisis of adolescence can, for Crisp, be termed 'the adolescent/family maturational crisis' (1979:

151). The struggle for independence and the development of a sexual identity can, for example, rekindle for the parents old, unresolved uncertainties about their own identities, their sexuality or their social confidence. Further, in some families where the parents have agreed to stay together only until their children grow up, adolescence threatens the very cohesion of the family (1977: 232; 1980: 66–9; Crisp *et al.*, 1980: 229). Such families have, in short, 'a (so far as the present problem is concerned) faulty way of life' (Crisp 1980: 137), and are often 'pathologically enmeshed and on the defensive against the outside world and its turmoil' (1983a: 857). These 'faulty' families can then produce a shy, timid and dependent child for whom growing up becomes a process so filled with anxiety that it is avoided in anorexia.

It can, however, be a purely individual pathology which makes a girl anorexic. She may have a 'major personality immaturity' (1980: 65), very low self-esteem, be especially shy or compliant or sexually insecure (1970b: 494; 1974: 526), or have 'major psychological developmental defects and an absence of other defense mechanisms' (Crisp *et al.*, 1977: 62–3). This individual psychological vulnerability may be exacerbated by an earlier than usual puberty, but in any case the pre-anorexic girl feels that she is incapable of becoming a competent adult, and her anxiety is such that she retains only 'a marginal or borderline sense of the self . . . predominantly in terms of shape' (Crisp, 1980: 55, 35; see also 1970a: 16; 1970b: 463). Food is avoided and comes to be 'hated and feared' because of its association with psychosexual growth, and the anorexic flight back into childhood begins (1970b: 454).

Crisp's explanation of anorexia logically results in a two-pronged treatment strategy. First, it is essential that the adolescent regains enough weight to tip her over the point at which hormonal development will be 'switched on', for she must actually reach pubertal weight in order to re-experience sexuality and get back in touch with 'her more natural psychological self' (1980: 140, 84–5, 103; Crisp and Fransella, 1979: 80). As well as this 're-exposure to the phobic situation', psychotherapy must help her to adjust better to and engage with adult life (Crisp, 1967: 716; 1980: preface). Autonomy, healthy independence and a sense of mastery over her destiny, plus the recognition that her feelings and needs are aspects of her personality that others value, can all be developed through a psychotherapeutic relationship in which the therapist fills a 'parental protective role', providing the secure interpersonal relationship that is necessary for adolescent development and has in all likelihood been missing (1967: 716; 1980: 142–7; 1983b).

CRITIQUE OF CRISP

Crisp's work on anorexia is extremely influential; he has, in fact, been the major British authority for the past three decades. Why, then, do I find his work so disappointing?

First, of course, as a psychiatrist Crisp assumes the fundamental psychiatric tenet that mental illness is 'soluble' at the individual level. *Why* anorexics should want or need to avoid the 'maturational challenge' and why *female* sexuality is especially problematical are questions answered by the definition of the anorexic girl as deficient. 'Normal' women, it is implied, face adulthood with equanimity, in spite of the fact that sexuality is more problematic for women. The socially created role of twentieth-century 'femininity' is so far naturalized as to disappear as an object of analysis. Thus Crisp cannot fully analyse what I would argue are *social* institutions – the role of women in bourgeois partriarchal societies, and feminine sexuality in particular here – because he views the process of becoming an adult as universal, ahistorical, natural and easy.

Further, the very notion of the individual is only partially understood, I would argue, when personality is seen as an inherent possession, and not as a creation of social forces. Thus the *class* distribution of anorexia nervosa, while noted, is left unexplained. Why we should find so many more deviant girls and faulty families among the middle classes remains an unanswered question. Related to this fundamental individualism intrinsic to psychiatric explanation is a biologically determinist view of human development specific to Crisp. In spite of brief references to social norms, such as the need for women to be slim and attractive, as specifically 'modern' (1974: 526), Crisp assumes a biologically determined and universal path to adulthood to which the only social and historical 'contributions' are moral rules and prohibitions – or the lack of them.

His notion of the adolescent personality's need to 'enlarge' to encompass sexuality seems to posit sexuality as a direct product of hormonal activity, only minimally affected by the need to be 'socially adaptive'. Further, he assumes the naturalness and universality of what I would argue is the *currently* dominant view of sexuality as naturally adult, heterosexual and genital, a sexuality which sociologists argue is the result of the channelling of a fluid human sexuality through the conduits of bourgeois and patriarchal values (1967: 714, 718; see Foucault, 1979; Weeks, 1986; Kitzinger, 1987). For Crisp there is a determinist connection between puberty, as marked by the pubertal weight threshold, and 'adolescent trauma' centring on selfhood and sexuality, a threshold which must be *personally* and *physically* experienced to be understood. This determinism does not allow for any consideration of how the social construction of adulthood and sexuality make sense of and give meaning to biological processes. It is biologism taken to the extreme to argue, as Crisp does, that it is the adolescent body which 'requires' the gender identity (1977: 232).

It would seem, therefore, that Crisp's theory of anorexia is based on an unquestioned acceptance of the norms of a bourgeois and patriarchal society as naturally human norms. Further, this perspective also leads to a lack of recognition of how these norms apply *differently* to women. Crisp aims to help the anorexic girl to 'a new freedom to explore and develop herself as a person' (1980: 147). Being a 'person' means being independent, feeling that you own your own body, having a greatly reduced concern with weight and shape and seeing yourself and your needs as valued by others (1980: 142–7; 1983b). I would – and will, in later chapters – question the extent to which any of this is tenable for *women*, for whom dependence, a devalued social role, concern with appearance and, crucially in anorexia, an 'open' concept of the body come as part and parcel of 'feminity'. Indeed, I will suggest that individualism itself, while being presented as an asexual, gender-neutral category, is thus presented *phallocentrically*, having been developed on a masculine model of the individual which is itself defined in opposition to femininity.

Finally, and following on from the above, I would argue that Crisp's focus on anorexia as an avoidance response fails to illuminate to any great degree the 'common-sense' categories on which his analysis is based. My own analysis will focus on the *social meanings* of food and the body, how these are created and maintained, how they are experienced specifically by women, how they are transformed in anorexia and how they change over time. This is an approach which the psychiatric understanding as a whole and

Crisp's version of it in particular precludes. When the conceptualization of the body is posited as a universal and basically unproblematic by-product of biological development, and when the only 'meaning' food has is limited to a simple association with growth and comfort (1981–2: 213), it is difficult to treat either as concepts deserving of real analysis.

In Crisp's analysis – as in most psychiatric work – what is deemed important is how anorexia nervosa is caused, *not* the meaning and significance of anorexic behaviour. After 'this is how it happens', explanation stops. This seems to me to be inadequate, both as analysis and, in Crisp's case, as causal explanation. Anorexic thinking and behaviour are not only deserving of analysis in their own right, but the question of how and why a process so fundamental as eating can be so radically transformed, if adequately answered, can explain not only the *anorexic* conceptualizations of food and the body, but will also illuminate other, more common conceptualizations and how these relate to wider social structures.

Further, I would argue that it is impossible to so definitively separate 'cause' and 'effect', as Crisp does when he argues that the root of anorexia is avoidance of adulthood, and it is not in itself an 'existentially fulfilling' experience (1983b). I would differentiate experience as existentially *fulfilling* and experience as existentially *meaningful*; Crisp does not and thus 'loses' the *meaning* of anorexia which, I would argue, ought to be basic to its analysis.

The 'new' or transformed meanings which food and the body come to have in anorexia will, in my own analysis, be compared with socially dominant ideas about food and the body in order to form what I hope will be a fuller explanation of anorexia than that offered by Crisp's biologism.

ROGER SLADE: THE INTERVENTION OF THE SOCIAL

Roger Slade's explanation of anorexia is constructed in the answer to two questions: how does the initial impetus to control food and lose weight arise; and how is it then maintained (Slade, 1984: 30)? In focusing on these questions Slade argues that anorexia is a two-stage process.

For Slade, the answer to his first question is to be found in social forces, in the combination of 'the ethics of body regulation' and the female gender role (ibid.: 147). He argues:

Belief in the value of hard work and consistent application is deeply engrained in our culture, as is the commitment to achievement through individual effort and the idea of deferring pleasures and gratifications until satisfactory ends have been attained. These are the values that were sanctified by Protestant sects in the early years of industrial capitalism.

(1984: 135)

Such values, Slade argues, emerge strongly in the middle-class family's commitment to personal achievement sought through hard work and disciplined self-control. Further, there is a strong connection between these values and body regulation, a link seen in the idea of sport as 'an ideal mode of training for the moral and social behaviour that is central to the highest concerns of society', and this concern creates the potential for *extreme* forms of bodily control, such as anorexia nervosa (ibid.: 138, 134–9).

Slade then goes on to suggest that when the 'ethics of body regulation', as described above, meet the female gender role anorexia becomes even more explicable, for it is the latter, in emphasizing compliance and the need for women to be physically attractive, which causes the pre-anorexic girl to be highly vulnerable to both familial pressures to succeed through personal effort, and social pressures to regulate her body through food control (ibid.: 144).

For women, the wider social values of assertiveness, independence, intellectual prowess and productivity conflict with the female role values of passivity, dependence, helplessness and being decorative. Most women adjust to this conflict by concentrating on 'feminine values', but the anorexic girl cannot do this as she is under strong pressure to succeed educationally, a pressure which is accentuated by the early lesson that assertiveness is inappropriate in women while being receptive to others' needs and demands is valued (ibid.: 174–9). The anorexic girl, Slade argues:

feels obliged to respond both in a way that is generally considered socially desirable for males, and in a way that is considered socially desirable for females. It is, paradoxically, because of her 'female' receptivity that she feels obliged to take on 'male' tasks.

(ibid.: 189–90)

Faced with this confusion, her family's expectations become her *personal* burden, and she feels increasingly unable to fulfil both those expectations and the social expectations of the female gender role (ibid.: 185). She is unable, faced with these conflicts, to develop a coherent sense of self. For Slade, decision-making allows the individual to influence events outside herself, and this sense of influential action is 'implicit in the idea of what it is to be a person' (ibid.: 166). He argues that:

> the sense of the self is generated in those things the person can do. The most characteristically human quality is not only the capacity to make decisions, but the capacity, in so doing to create one's own being.
>
> (ibid.: 166)

The anorexic girl's inability to act decisively prevents the development of 'a stable set of preferences . . .[or] core of personal values', and she therefore lacks a clear or enduring sense of self (ibid.: 167). It is in this context that slimming, a common activity among teenage girls, assumes special significance for the anorexic. Food control is the one area of her life which seems to the anorexic girl to be amenable to her own controlling influence, and her success in this one area is what will eventually trap her into anorexia. Control of eating is reliable, does not involve other people, and becomes the only part of her life which is 'consistently and uncomplicatedly good' (ibid.: 160). Food control becomes for the anorexic girl 'a last-ditch attempt to retain her sense of self through effective action, however limited' (ibid.: 112). This, then, is 'Stage 1' of anorexia nervosa.

In 'Stage 2', Slade hypothesizes that the psychological consequences of starvation then work to change anorexia from a deliberate, conscious action into an 'externally' maintained trap, a state of being which escapes the individual's control. Once the effects of starvation on her thought processes become established, the anorexic girl is trapped 'in the grip of processes that run away with her' (ibid.: 12). What, then, are these processes?

Slade argues that starvation changes the way in which people think, and that these changes are just as predictable as are the physical changes of starvation. Reduction in the intake of food, it is suggested, produces a progressive decline in intellectual capacity. Instability in neural activity is caused by the effects of starvation which then make the conditions for the proper working of the brain unstable, and this instability results in the impairment of 'the highest mental function of reason and abstract thought' (ibid.: 70–1; 69). The capacity to engage in complex thinking is progressively diminished; the world is seen increasingly in terms of simple sets of categories – black and white, good and bad – with no intermediate stages. In short, Slade argues, thinking becomes *polarized*. Her restricted capacity for thinking means that food control becomes the anorexic's main preoccupation; in fact, she is *incapable* of being anything other than obsessed with food and weight. This state could, in principle, be viewed either as positive or negative, but because of the conflict and confusion which has characterized her pre-anorexic life, restricted thinking is experienced by the anorexic as a welcome withdrawal from day-to-day life. Furthermore, the high value that she places on control of food and her body also act to 'set' the anorexic girl to interpret the effects of starvation in a positive way (ibid.: 72–8).

When weight falls to between 70 and 80 per cent of average expected body weight this 'characteristic anorexic way of thinking' occurs, and it is here, Slade argues, that the 'whirlpool effect' takes over:

> by severely reducing the amount of food she eats, the anorexic simplifies her thinking. As her style of thinking changes, her decision not to eat is reinforced. As a consequence of this she grows even thinner and the cycle continues. The more emaciated she becomes the easier it is for her to make the decision not to eat. So she spirals downward.
>
> (ibid.: 77, 74)

CRITIQUE OF SLADE

Slade's analysis raises a number of valid and interesting points. The explanation in terms of social forces of the initial stage of anorexia is useful, especially when compared to the biological determinism of Crisp. However, it is in explanations of this type that the need for a *fully* sociological analysis of anorexia is, I would argue, most clearly evident. Slade asserts a significant 'input' into individual psychology of cultural values – and indeed, much psychiatric writing on anorexia follows this line – but these explanations should not be seen as *sociological*. They represent, I would argue, little more than a 'flirtation' with the concept of socially constructed individuality, and in the final analysis revert to 'individual pathology' as the fundamental cause of mental illness.

In Slade's analysis, the effect of social forces is 'grafted on' to the individualist and psychologistic understanding of personality as a unique individual possession. In this perspective culture is external to the individual and its 'external' effects can thus only be secondary. As Slade puts it, the *extreme* behaviour of the anorexic makes it clear that 'the manner in which she behaves must be explained, not in terms of culture, but in terms of individual psychological constraints' (ibid.: 154). Thus, in spite of the at-first-glance promising, even near-Marxist argument that the self is created through activity, it later becomes clear that for Slade this activity is itself not socially constructed but individualistic.

Furthermore, his conception of the relationship of social forces and the individual is *determinist*. Part of the ultimate rejection of the notion of 'social' causation for Slade (and others) is that not *all* young middle-class women, subject to more or less the same social and familial pressures, become anorexic. This assumes a remorseless cause and effect relation between circumstances and behaviour, and does not see that circumstances limit but do not determine the *range* of possible behaviours. Women respond to the pressures of a patriarchal and capitalist society in a variety of ways of which, as I will argue, the anorexic response is one.

There is a second determinist element in Slade's analysis. Although in my own analysis of anorexia I will argue that there are good reasons to see anorexia as a 'two-stage' process, the organicist explanation of 'starvation stage' anorexia which Slade offers is, I would argue, far from sufficient. Slade suggests that in a culture which values bodily control the psychological effects of starvation on the brain can be interpreted positively; however, in themselves these effects are in no sense socially constructed. Reduced capacity in the 'higher' functions of the brain is posited as having a single and unitary cause – the effect of starvation on the hypothalamus – which determines outcome. As Slade himself points out, the hypothalamus remains poorly understood; thus, his argument remains problematic on the organic level alone (ibid.: 34).[3] Further, he does not adequately argue the case for mental *incapacity* in Stage 2 anorexia; it could, alternatively, be argued that it is not the *ability* to engage in 'complex' thinking but the *will* to do so which is lacking. Here, Slade is again operating on a simplistic 'cause and effect' model of experience. Hypothalamic malfunction determines reduced thinking; bodily/food control already exists; therefore the anorexic can only think about food. The *meanings* food comes to have in anorexia, *how* the anorexic girl makes sense of her experience of eating does not need to be explained. If, however, we adopt an approach which sees the structure and concepts of thought as socially constructed in a dialectical, not a determinist, relationship with physiological states which them- selves must be socially interpreted in order to be meaningful, the explanation of 'Stage 2' anorexia should *begin* at the point where Slade's analysis ends.

Further, the meanings of food, eating and the body can in this perspective be analysed as social products rather than naturalized and accepted as completely unproblematical and existing only in one 'natural' form. (See, for example, Slade's argument that ideas about food are the only ideas which are not 'conflicting and confused' (ibid.: 173).) This would then allow anorexic food con- trol to become the *real* object of analysis. In later chapters I will argue that in 'starvation stage' anorexia food comes to be repre- sentative of all 'external' influences on and connections with the inner self and that it is for *this* reason that food control dominates 'anorexic thinking'. Here, food rituals – what is allowed entry to, and kept in, the body – are used, I will argue, to maintain a rigid psychic boundary around the self. The social meanings of food are *transformed* in anorexia into *alternative*, not merely 'reduced' or 'deficient', categorizations.

In short, then, a fully sociological analysis of anorexia would see the social construction of physiological states, and the alternative constructions of anorexia as the objects of analysis. It is not only that anorexia *exists*, but what it means and how it is experienced that is important. This perspective further has the advantage of seeing the anorexic girl as actively creative *of*, and not simply passively controlled *by* her bodily functions.

HILDE BRUCH: OVER-COMPLIANT DAUGHTERS

For Hilde Bruch, anorexia nervosa is 'the relentless pursuit of thinness' (Bruch, 1974: 224; 1978: x). In anorexia, self-denial and discipline are seen as the highest virtues, satisfying needs and desires as 'shameful self-indulgence' (1974: 268; 1978: x). Self- denial in the form of food control is secondary to a struggle for identity and selfhood; food control and being able to stand hunger, and indeed training herself to *value* hunger, give to the anorexic woman 'the feeling of a personality core' which she would otherwise lack. Thinness becomes her 'supreme achievement', the purpose of her existence (1978: x, 4–7). The essence of anorexia, for Bruch, is therefore not centred on food and weight – these are respectively a *method* and a *proof*. The anorexic *uses* starvation and the domination of bodily desires in her search for control, identity and competence, and uses the resulting thinness as the sign that her control is effective (1974: 252).

Bruch argues that three areas of 'disturbed psychological functioning' lie at the heart of anorexia (1970: 12–15; 1974: 252–6; 1978: x). First, the anorexic woman has a 'near delusional' body-image. She will consistently claim that she is not, in fact, thin, and overestimates both her own size, others' sizes, and abstract distances (1978: 46, 78). Second, anorexic women cannot correctly identify bodily stimuli, especially hunger. Awareness of hunger, Bruch argues, is not instinctive, that is, is not 'innate biological knowledge'. Therefore *learning* is necessary for hunger – and indeed all biological needs – to become 'organized into recognizable patterns' (1969: 93).

This process of learning, for the 'pre-anorexic', is to be sought in childhood experience where the child's needs are not correctly recognized by the mother, who feeds the child to her own schedule, not on demand, and offers inappropriate responses to 'child-initiated cues' – be those responses 'neglectful, oversolicitous, inhibiting or indiscriminately permissive' (1969: 99). The child thus grows up with no sense of being in control of, or even properly recognizing, her own bodily sensations. Because of this, the anorexic woman suffers from a profound sense of ineffectiveness. She feels that she is living her life in accordance with the demands of others, and has no confidence that she could do otherwise (1971: 241; 1975: 161; 1977: 4; 1980: 170). Bruch argues that if the mother, and not the child, has constantly initiated action 'her child may grow up living entirely by responding to others . . . he will never know that thoughts, feelings or actions originating in him can be effective' (1969: 53). Bruch cites the case of 'Sharon', who dated the real onset of her anorexia to a class in literature where a poem had a profound effect on her, revealing that she had no idea how to be 'the captain of my soul' and 'the master of my fate' (1974: 263).

The anorexic girl, then, arrives at adolescence with serious 'ego deficiencies'. She experiences her life as being under the control of others, and she has no coherent or self-directed identity (1969: 100; 1974: 285, 376). Adolescence, however, is a time when self-reliant independence must be developed, and it is at this point when 'positive self-assertion becomes unavoidable . . .[and] the severe deficiencies in the core personality become apparent' (1970: 15). The anorexic's ego simply cannot cope with the demands of adolescence and she withdraws into her own body as the only place she feels she can control and into food control as an attempt to undo the bodily aspects of adolescence (1980: 170).

How, then, do these 'ego deficiences' arise? Bruch argues that the cause is to be found in 'abnormal patterns of family interaction' (1978: 106). In the family histories of her anorexic patients the consistent description of the anorexic daughter is of the perfect child – well-behaved, academically successful and compliant. Parents often told her that 'the miserable, angry and desperate patient had been the best, sweetest, most obedient and most cooperative child ever' (1978: 38). But behind this rosy picture, Bruch argues, is a failure on the part of the parents to transmit to their daughters a sense of competence and self-value. The child is valued not as an individual in her own right, but as someone whose success would compensate for the *parents'* 'concealed dissatisfactions and disappointments', especially those of the mother, who is often a 'frustrated career woman' (1970: 20; 1971: 245). As such, then, the daughter is given no opportunity for 'constructive self-assertion' (1978: 37). In the face of these excessive demands, and cloaked by her over-conformity, the anorexic-to-be suffers great anxiety, constantly concerned with being unable to live up to her parents' expectations and thus losing their love. In spite of the fact that they were treated as 'special', they felt 'undeserving, unworthy and ungrateful', both burdened by and incapable of achieving the success expected (1978: 39). Frequently, they describe themselves as 'blanks' (1978: 48).

Further, Bruch argues that anorexic girls had always resented this parental over-control, and anorexia should be seen as part of the unacknowledged struggle for independence between them and their parents. In short, 'they would rather starve themselves than continue a life of accommodation' (1977: 1; 2–3).

Anorexia can be seen to serve two functions in this analysis. It is part of a very delayed attempt at independence, and is also an attempt to impose a *personal* control over the body. However, because of the underlying and continuing deficient awareness of and control over bodily sensations, food control *itself* 'gets away' from them, and is experienced as an *external* control, as a 'mysterious force that invades them or directs their behaviour' (1978: 55). Anorexia as an adaptational pattern does not work (1970: 21). Therapy, therefore, should aim to help the anorexic to develop a strong self-concept and identity in which she feels herself capable of self-directed action, self-regulation of her needs and desires, and of owning her own body. She must be shown that it is *wrong* to feel ineffective and devalued, and that her own needs, thoughts and actions are of 'fundamental importance' (1974: 63). Thus, and only thus, will the 'golden cage' of anorexia be opened.

CRITIQUE OF BRUCH

It would seem, therefore, that for Bruch anorexia nervosa is best understood as a kind of hysteria or conversion disorder, in which the physical symptoms are meaningful not so much in themselves, but as the manifestations of an underlying psychological disorder – the lack of a fully-developed sense of self. And following the psychoanalytic tradition, the causes of this disorder are located in infantile and childhood experience, centred on the family unit.

Thus anorexia, it is argued, is fundamentally a disorder of the self, rather than a disorder of weight, food or appetite. This perspective leads Bruch virtually to ignore the possible role and meanings of food and the body in anorexia. Both are taken as relatively unproblematic; food is simply 'available' to be used in the struggle for selfhood and control, and its possible *social* significance is ignored, apart from a brief consideration of increased food intake as the 'fuel' of the pubertal processes, the reduction of which, as in Crisp's analysis, is used in an attempt to 'undo' physical maturity (1978: 59).

Further, the significance of the choice of the body and the manipulation of body-weight as the main arena of anorexic behaviour also remains an uninvestigated area of Bruch's thesis, thinness being, for Bruch, no more than 'evidence' that anorexic control is working. In spite of noting media pressures on young women to be slim, the real significance of the anorexic body is, for Bruch, minimal. What having an adult female body *means* in a culture which simultaneously eroticizes, degrades and devalues both women and their bodies, and how the transformation of the formally asexual child's body into the ambiguous icon of the female body is *experienced*, are questions which are simply left unasked as the focus of analysis is exclusively on inferred underlying psychological forces. And while in my own analysis I too will focus, as Bruch does, on issues of selfhood and control, I see it as one of the main benefits of a *sociological* analysis of anorexia that both the 'underlying' and the 'surface' facets of anorexia can become *full* objects of investigation, phenomena whose meanings and interconnections are not assumed to be either prosaic or already understood.

That having been said, what ought we to make of Bruch's analysis of the underlying psychological causation of anorexia? For Bruch, as we have seen, anorexia is in essence a struggle for identity and selfhood, precipitated when the onset of puberty demands a move to independence and maturity of which the 'core-less' personality of the anorexic is incapable. Here, I would argue, Bruch builds her theory on an unexplicated and assumed understanding of individual personality development which is both ahistorical, and while *formally* gender-neutral, is in fact a *masculine* model of development. Thus her understanding of anorexia is severely limited.

Bruch's analysis of anorexia rests on the concept of the 'integrated body-self', or 'ego synthesis', in which the body and the self are experienced as a unity, and which is the normal outcome of personality development (1969: 102, 105). In short, in normal development 'a child learns to think of body and self as occupying the same space and forming a single functioning unit, separate from the units around him' (1969: 103). This process centres on the infant's demarcation of his own 'body-self' from the primary object, the mother, a process which, as we have seen, is posited as being inadequately achieved in anorexia (1969: 105).

Thus, one aim of therapy in anorexia is to 'clarify the disturbed interactional patterns so that the child can develop controls from within and become capable of experiencing himself as self-directed and as owning his body' (1971: 247). The body-self, then, is conceived of as a self-contained system of integrated sensations, needs and desires which is fundamentally separate from the environment, and in which both the body as a whole and its needs and sensations are experienced as self-directed and *owned* by the self. The self-contained system must be just that – a *system*, and not 'a loose organization of [need] patterns and associated desires' in which incoherence makes *disintegration* an ever-present possibility (1969: 100).

Bruch's body-self concept is, as I think the summary above shows, fundamentally confused. The 'integrated' body-self can only be integrated to a very limited degree (i.e. spatially) if the body and its needs and desires are seen to be 'owned' by the self. Bruch seems to be working with two not entirely reconcilable notions here; first, of the ideal healthy individual who experiences the physical as so entirely 'natural' and unproblematic that s/he sees him/herself as a 'physical' entity; and second, of the older notion of the self as separate from and *owning*, although contained in, the body.

As well as this conceptual confusion the problems of analysing a feminine experience through a masculine model of the individual cause the analysis to crack further under scrutiny. In a culture in which the gender division is a basic organizational category, there are, I would argue, fundamental differences in masculine and feminine 'selfhood' which patriarchal psychiatry obscures by positing a gender-neutral model of the individual.

Independence, separateness and being self-contained, both physically and psychologically, are, I will later argue, characteristic of the 'ideal *man*' not the ideal woman. The concept of absolute bodily integrity and separation is an unattainable ideal for women, as is that independence which rests on a conception of one's own needs, thoughts and actions as of 'fundamental importance' (1974: 63). For women, physical and psychological and emotional openness is central. The dominant notion of the individual in a patriarchal culture coexists with an ideal of feminine *receptiveness*, both physical/sexual and psychological/emotional, which relates to the role of women as 'complementary' to, and defined in relation to men. This receptiveness, however, is enforced but not valued. With a dominant concept of individuality in which separateness and bodily and psychological 'integrity' are central, receptiveness means weakness, vulnerability and incompletion and is regarded with a mixture of fear, fascination and disgust.

Thus, I would argue, Bruch's uncritical acceptance of a 'gender-neutral' concept of the individual, in terms of both body and psyche, seriously limits her understanding of anorexia, leading her to analyse feminine receptiveness in anorexia, not as a central part of being an adequate woman in a patriarchal culture, but as 'ego deficiency' arising from an 'abnormal' family (1974: 78; 1978:

101). She either simply does not, or *chooses* not to see that 'separate-unit' psychology is far from being the gender-neutral standard of her theory. Her only 'solution' is an attempt through therapy to help women better integrate the conflicting demands of individualism and receptiveness, an integration which must take place *without* exposing the confusion and conflicts of these demands to the light of day, lest the goal of perfect adaptation to the demands of the culture be seen as being, for women, an impossible goal.

Furthermore, the idea of the individual as a self-contained system is treated in Bruch's work as universally applicable. Bourgeois individualism, as well as being an essentially masculine concept, is also, I will argue, a *historical* concept. I hope to demonstrate later, through a comparison of the bourgeois concept of the individualized and atomized body with the medieval concept of the fluid and open body of the people, that conceptualizations of the body are not static but reflect and change with changes in the wider social structure. Similarly, the concept of the individual itself is also a historical concept, and is linked to conceptualizations of the body.

I would like to conclude by noting some more minor confusions in Bruch's analysis of anorexia. The idea of 'disturbed psychological functioning' – that anorexics do not properly recognize hunger, and do not 'see' that they are thin – is contradicted by the argument, which we can also find in Bruch's work, that being able to 'stand' hunger and sustain extreme thinness are used by the anorexic as a sign of her mastery of her body (1974: 41; 1978: x). This confusion results from her attempt to introduce elements of biological causation into an essentially intrapsychic explanation, but it does not fundamentally affect the argument that anorexia nervosa is a struggle for selfhood through bodily control, although the rejection of biological 'drivenness' would force her to analyse anorexia as a more active and chosen process.

Further, Bruch's inability to perceive how therapy, which she sees as wholly beneficial, could be seen by the anorexic woman as a threat to her precious and precarious control, leads her, like Crisp and Slade, to exclude the possibility that 'rigid' thought and behaviour patterns could be adopted as a defence against therapeutic attack. She therefore argues not that the anorexic *must* be rigid in what she will and will not allow in order to maintain her anorexia, but that she is – as Slade argues – *incapable* of any more flexible thinking, an assertion for which there is both little evidence and possible alternative explanations. It would seem, therefore, that the most central and interesting questions raised by anorexia remain unasked and unanswered in Bruch's thesis. Why anorexia is so overwhelmingly a *feminine* experience is an issue which cannot be approached more than superficially – in brief references to 'media pressures' which seem to exist independently of the real world – if a phallocentric model of individuality is to be maintained. And the *meanings* of food and the body, both in society as a whole and specifically in anorexia cannot be analysed if they are seen as, respectively, 'natural' and unproblematical, and ahistorical and gender-neutral phenomena. However, although I have suggested that Bruch uses an oversimplified separation of the physical and the psychic in her analysis and overconcentrates on the latter, I accept the centrality of control in anorexia, and also see as significant, although for different reasons, diffuse 'ego boundaries', and her focus on separation and boundaries in general. This I hope to explain further and better in my own analysis of anorexia.

MARA SELVINI PALAZZOLI: THE OBJECT BODY

The work of the Italian psychoanalyst Mara Selvini Palazzoli is similar to Hilde Bruch's analysis in many ways. Indeed, in her earliest writings, Palazzoli analysed anorexia as a disturbance of 'body cognition', an inability to identify or distinguish between different inner states, impulses and desires. This, she argues, arises out of a disturbed and confusing relationship with a mother 'impervious' to the child's needs, which causes an inadequate perception of bodily needs when the child becomes an adult. This is essentially Bruch's thesis, and both agree that anorexia is deficient functioning caused by a faulty relationship to the body as 'the basic source of experience' (Palazzoli, 1967: 312; 1969: 256).

Palazzoli, however, went on to develop her understanding of anorexia further in her *Self-starvation: From the Intrapsychic to the Transpersonal Approach to Anorexia Nervosa* (1974). As the title shows, while Palazzoli was developing her analysis she was 'converted' to family therapy, which sees the illness of an individual family member as the outcome of family 'malfunctions', with the family seen as a 'homeostatic unit', that is, a self-regulating entity based on its own rules (ibid.: 196–200, 228–31). While both her intrapsychic and intrafamilial explanations of anorexia have their problems, in her intrapsychic manifestation Palazzoli offers some interesting and enlightening notions on the meaning of food and the body in anorexia, and it is on these that I would like to focus.

Palazzoli starts her explanation of anorexia by using object-relations theory. She argues that the child's original experience with the primary object – the mother, or food equalling mother – is a 'corporeal-incorporative' experience; the infant's inability to distinguish himself and the object means that incorporation is the only way he *can* relate to it. Now, the object has both positive (pleasureable, nurturing) and negative (unpleasant, rejecting) aspects, and while the normal child in a satisfactory relationship with his mother will gradually learn to perceive his body as a separate whole, existing *outside* the maternal object, and therefore not as the source of 'bad' sensations, in 'psychopathological' development:

> the condition of being 'outside' is realized in part only. Most of the 'bad' experiences of his own body, which the child has met during the incorporative, primary narcissistic, phase of his object relationships, remain immured inside his body.
>
> (ibid.: 84–5)

It is, therefore, the body itself that the anorexic fears:

> the body of the anorexic does not merely *contain* the bad object but . . . *is* the bad object . . . the body is experienced as having all the features of the primary object as it was perceived in a situation of oral helplessness: all-powerful, indestructible, self-sufficient, growing and threatening . . . there is an unconscious feeling that the object is far too strong to be destroyed.
>
> (ibid.: 87)

The body is therefore equated with the negative and overpowering aspects of the incorporated object.

Puberty, then, is the crucial moment in anorexia, when those negative aspects of the object are separated from the ego in order that they can be opposed. Three processes are at work here. First, it is at this time that an independent personal identity must be formed, and the anorexic woman, because of the faulty early learning which has made her dependent and compliant, feels herself unequal to this challenge and the ensuing trauma 'reactivates the overwhelming sense of helplessness experienced during the infantile period' (ibid.: 89; 56; 77). Thus far, Palazzoli follows

Bruch. From here on, however, she moves onto new ground, using
Arieti's concept of 'concretization':

> In the Freudian view, phobia is a form of displacement. Thus
> while little Hans was afraid of his father, his neurosis displaced
> that fear on to horses. According to Freud, such displacement
> serves to conceal a sexual threat, and therefore becomes sym-
> bolic of what it replaces . . . the displacement is not necessarily
> from one object to another. What happens is not so much a
> displacement as a concretization. The patient lives in fear of
> vague and intangible threats that he may find difficult to define
> or that he refuses to recognize . . . In patients suffering from
> serious phobias the psychiatrist can easily recognize the concre-
> tization of a more general anxiety-producing situation . . . In
> my view, phobia is the expression of a general psychopathologi-
> cal principle, namely that *whatever cannot be borne abstractly*
> *because it generates too much anxiety . . . will eventually be concretized.*
> This concretization of concepts and intuitions is not simply a
> reduction of the abstract to the concrete level. . . . but an active
> process, i.e. an active translation of the abstract into the con-
> crete.
>
> (quoted ibid.: 148–9)

It is, therefore, at puberty that what the pre-anorexic girl fears and
finds threatening becomes 'concretized' into the newly developed
adult female body as a phobic object. The second process of
'anorexic puberty', then, is the transformation of the earlier *psychic*
incorporation of the object into a *physically concrete* incorporation:

> because of the development of the breasts and other feminine
> curves, the body is experienced *concretely* as the maternal object
> . . . [and] . . . the patient considers and experiences her body as
> one great incorporated object which overpowers her and forces
> a passive role upon her.
>
> (ibid.: 90)

The pre-pubertal sense of the bad object as invincible is also
transformed at puberty, for now that the bad object is concretely
equated by the anorexic with *her* body, it is newly amenable to the
active aggression of starvation. However, because the body, like
the bad object, is *fascinating* as well as overpowering, it cannot be
simply abandoned but must be kept under control and its growth
prevented (ibid.: 90–2).

Third, it is at puberty that what Palazzoli terms the 'passive-receptive aspect of feminine life' is first experienced (ibid.: 70). Not only is the physical aspect of puberty experienced as 'a sudden, mysterious and humiliating bodily happening over which the poor girl has no control', but the adult female body must be accepted as 'an essentially receptive-passive object' (ibid.: 69–70). Palazzoli argues thus:

> the adolescent girl . . . experiences her feminine sexuality in a passive and receptive way: she is exposed to lewd looks, subjected to menstruation, about to be penetrated in sexual embraces, to be invaded by the foetus, to be suckled by a child.
> (ibid.: 70)

The new woman's body as a whole, then, also comes to represent concretely this passivity and receptiveness, and is rejected/controlled not only as the concrete manifestation of the negative and overpowering aspects of the maternal object, but also as the concrete manifestation of receptiveness/passivity. The anorexic girl is attempting to become an autonomous adult 'by rejecting those aspects of feminine corporeality that conjure up the terrifying vista of turning into a succubus and passive vessel' (ibid.: 72).

The body, then, is ambiguously experienced as both alien and persecuting, in its status as phobic object in identification with the bad object and with feminine receptiveness, *and* as owned, and thus amenable to manipulation (ibid.: 93, 63–4). Eating never having been experienced as *personally* controllable, food represents losing control as well as, as a material substance, bodily increase. Thus body growth is perceived as taking place at the expense of the ego or self, which has identified itself 'with an ideal that is a desexualised, acarnal and essentially powerful image', 'a psychotic ideal of acorporeality', an ideal which hunger threatens (ibid.: 90; 150–1; 86–7).

For Palazzoli the failure to perceive bodily signals which originally, following Bruch, she saw as central to the explanation of anorexia, is in the end downgraded. She concludes that a failure to perceive bodily signals, especially hunger, is consequent upon the rejection of the body as phobic object, and that it is the latter, not the former, which is the primary anorexic process. The anorexic girl, then, experiences stasis: she must contain and control the body without destroying it; she must continue to live but she cannot grow.

CRITIQUE OF PALAZZOLI

Palazzoli, then, while ostensibly following the Bruch line, in fact branches off into areas Bruch leaves unanalysed. For me, the most exciting part of her work is her reconstruction of some of the ways in which the transformation of the 'asexual' child's body into the eroticized and degraded adult female body can be experienced, that is, what *meanings* the adult female body can come to have.

However, once again the focus on the domestic and the familial as the centre of the female universe limits the possibilities of analysis, and leaves unexplored the *social* construction of meaning. The 'bad object' from this perspective is, literally, the mother – and in more ways than one. For Palazzoli, as for Bruch, the root 'cause' of anorexia is maternal failing – the mother fails to teach her child that she is a separate and autonomous individual, and so the girl, at adolescence, is unable to cope with the social demands to begin to become an independent adult. Once again, the underlying assumption* is that a 'good' mother will produce a 'good' or 'normal' – that is, non-anorexic – daughter; and that, consequently, it is the deviance of the individual, and not the conflicting demands of the culture that explain anorexia.

The 'psychiatric ideology', to use Penfold and Walker's term, *must* see the masculine bourgeois ideal of the autonomous and separate individual as 'natural', and therefore its attainment as possible for all but the deviant few, for if it does not it risks seeing psychologically autonomous individuality as a socially created and historically specific concept rather than as the universal outcome of all 'normal' development.

Broadly the same criticisms, then, can be levelled at Palazzoli's work as were applied to Bruch's, centring on the assumption that becoming a woman is psychologically unproblematic within the 'normal' family. However, what is *different* about Palazzoli's work is its continual threat to break out of its limits, a threat which gives her analysis the potential to be used in non-psychiatric explanations. Her explanation of how the adult female body is experienced contains a rich vein of ideas; I'd like to focus on two.

First, Palazzoli argues that the newly developing adult female body is experienced by the adolescent girl as 'all-powerful, inde-structible, self-sufficient, growing and threatening' in its association with the 'bad' aspects of the primary object (1974: 87). However, *simultaneously* the body is 'an essentially receptive-passive object' which is irremediably open and vulnerable to invasion (ibid.: 69–70). Palazzoli explains the overwhelming, powerful aspect of the female body as created through the association between the body-as-phobic-object and the infant's perception of the mother, and the passive, vulnerable aspect as a direct consequence of anatomical reality.

Both conceptualizations of the female body are, however, open to alternative and *wider* explanations. The understanding of female power as threatening and overwhelming has more behind it, I would argue, than simply literal description of the mother–child relationship. The 'threat' of *maternal* power is a threat to the child's separation from the mother, a threat to individual autonomy and therefore a threat which can only exist in the context of an individualized psychology. Further, I would argue that 'maternal' power should not be separated from feminine power as a whole. Fear of the suppressed power of an oppressed group can be shared by both oppressor and oppressed, and fear of the contained power of women is reflected in the conceptualization of female power as a threatening and encroaching force, threatening and encroaching on patriarchal power and patriarchal order, threatening to overwhelm and destroy 'femininity', that is, women's acquiescence to patriarchy. Thus, I would argue, one aspect of the social conceptualization of womanhood is of contained power, and this is a concept which, although given special emphasis and transformative attention in anorexia, is 'available' as a social meaning to *all* women, not merely to those suffering from a 'deviant' upbringing.

Further, I would argue that feminine 'openness' is not simply anatomical. The image of the female body arises not directly from physical reality but is created in ideology and material practice. It is not the body itself which makes women 'passive vessels', but how that body is *socially constructed*. The idea of the female body as open and incomplete is, as I will argue later, a reflection of women's position as 'secondary' to men and therefore incomplete. As I have suggested, the idea of an atomized and psychically coherent self is a masculine ideal, and the notion of women as physically open must be seen in relation to the psychological receptiveness which is a central tenet of the feminine role in patriarchy.

Therefore, while I would reject Palazzoli's domestic and anatomical explanations for the degraded modern concept of the female body – in anorexia, as in the wider society – as simultaneously threatening and open to invasion, I do see these concepts as central to any adequate analysis of anorexia, which sees anorexia both as an attempt to control and contain feminine desire *and* as a protection against the fear of psychological invasion. In later chapters, then, I will explore in greater depth the ideas about the female body which Palazzoli so interestingly raises here.

CONCLUSION

Crisp, Slade, Bruch and Palazzoli, then, while offering varying analyses of anorexia, share in common an individualist slant which sees anorexia as, in the last instance, a problem of individual deviance or deficiency. Thus, the culture which produces anorexia is normalized out of their analyses. This, for the feminist as for the sociologist, is profoundly unsatisfactory, especially in its down-grading of the role of cultural meanings in anorexia.

Two points, however, arise from this chapter. First, desire is obliquely or directly present in the work of all four writers; anorexic women are understood as unable to accept their desires and needs as 'normal', and are thus unable to act to fulfil them. It is this inability which accounts for their defective sense of self. Desire, thus, is central to being a person. Second, it is suggested that anorexic women need to be 'retrained' to independence and autonomy. Dependence, which is central to femininity, is thus a problem in anorexia.

In the psychiatric ideology, the desiring self and the dependent woman simply exist, requiring no analysis. For the feminist and the sociologist their isolation in psychiatric analysis is the starting-point rather than the end of theory. In Part III, dependence and desire will form central axes of my own analysis of anorexia. In the following chapter I will discuss the work of three feminist writers on anorexia, tracing their analyses of dependence and desire in the light of feminist theory's critique of the concept of natural femininity. We would expect feminist analyses to locate anorexia in patriarchally constructed femininity rather than seeing it as an incomplete development of gender-neutral individuality. It is to the question of how far this expectation is fulfilled that we now turn.

Chapter 3

Women's oppression
Feminist explanations of anorexia

Feminist work on anorexia is better known than it is plentiful. In Britain, Marilyn Lawrence's book *The Anorexic Experience* was for several years the only major feminist work on anorexia (Lawrence, 1984a). In 1986, however, Susie Orbach's *Hunger Strike* was published. Susie Orbach is perhaps best known for her bestseller *Fat is a Feminist Issue*, her work at the Women's Therapy Centre in London, and her writings, with Luise Eichenbaum, on female psychology (Orbach, 1978; Orbach and Eichenbaum, 1983). In America Kim Chernin has developed a feminist perspective on the issue of body-size in her books *Womansize: The Tyranny of Slenderness* and *The Hungry Self: Women, Eating and Identity* (Chernin, 1983; 1986). Both Chernin and Orbach, then, developed their interest in anorexia out of a concern with women, eating and body-size as a whole, while Lawrence worked with anorexic women as a psychiatric social worker.

All three writers are critical of orthodox psychiatric explanations of anorexia, and of psychiatric treatment of anorexia. A feminist perspective leads them to analyse anorexia as an issue of women's position in a patriarchal culture. What I hope to show in this chapter, however, are the limitations of constructing feminist explanations of anorexia without a *fully* sociological perspective. While a commitment to feminism pushes these theories towards seeing 'psychology' as a changeable, and therefore social and historical phenomenon, the underlying retention of the bourgeois concept of 'human nature' constrains the extent to which feminism can overturn psychiatric ideology. The fundamental assumption that an individualized self exists a priori and in ungendered form, and that the social structure prevents women from fully developing this self crucially limits the analysis. What results is the *addition* of a feminist view to underlying bourgeois patriarchal models of the self and of the body, rather than a feminist *critique* of those concepts.

This, I will argue, creates a subliminal tension in these analyses, which Orbach and Lawrence deal with by suggesting a 'two-stage' solution to anorexia – immediate individual therapy plus long-term social change – and which Chernin deals with by a call to value 'innate' 'female' qualities. Obviously, and especially with Orbach and Lawrence, their aim is therapy and mine is not, so I can afford to be more pessimistic about the prospects of individualist solutions. What this book argues is that in a bourgeois and patriarchal culture women *cannot* attain the socially valued self, since that self, far from being gender-neutral, is in fact masculine, and depends for its existence on an opposition with the receptive feminine self. Thus, I will argue that the central issue of anorexia is not how women are prevented from fully developing a self which exists in embryonic form, but rather a struggle between the ideologies of individualism and femininity.

In spite of these limitations, however, Orbach and Lawrence provide compelling analyses of anorexia which, from the sociological perspective, are a significant improvement on orthodox psychiatric and psychological theories. Orbach and Lawrence engage with the concepts of control and bodily and psychic boundaries which we saw in the work of Bruch and Palazzoli, but engage with them as feminists. Thus, they provide much more satisfactory analyses of the meanings of these concepts for women in a patriarchal culture, and of their centrality in anorexia. Chernin, although presenting the sociologist with more problems in her analysis of anorexia, does raise the vital issue of guilt, and makes some interesting points about anorexia as ritual behaviour.

This chapter, then, exists as much to pick up on what feminists have argued are the central issues in anorexia as to offer a sociological critique of current feminist work, and the issues of control, boundaries, guilt and ritual which we find in the work of the three feminist writers will form central axes of my own analysis of anorexia.

KIM CHERNIN: MOTHERS AND DAUGHTERS 1

In *Womansize: The Tyranny of Slenderness* Kim Chernin looked at cultural pressures on women to achieve and maintain a single socially approved body-shape (Chernin, 1983). In *The Hungry Self: Women, Eating and Identity* she goes on to look at eating disorders, including anorexia, arguing that they should be seen not simply as illnesses but as a 'hidden struggle for self-development' (Chernin, 1986: xiv).

Chernin analyses the issue of women and eating disorders by looking in turn at four main areas: the search for 'identity' and selfhood; the daughter's struggle to separate from the mother; food and its meanings for women; and the concept of the 'rite of passage'. Obsession with food is, for Chernin, a failed rite of passage. She argues:

> a troubled relationship to food frequently hides a serious problem with female identity in an age when women are invited by social circumstance and individual inclination to extend the traditional idea of what it means to be a woman.
>
> (ibid.: xi)

Extending tradition is, however, far from easy, and it is the ambivalence and guilt which women feel as they move into 'the male sphere of self-development and social power' which diverts the desire for change and self-development into the stagnation and misery of eating disorders (ibid.: xiv). Chernin then concludes with ideas on how the struggle for female identity could be less destructively effected.

She argues that it is only recently that women have claimed the right to participate in the public sphere in such large numbers (ibid.: xii). She writes:

> We are a unique generation of women – the first in history to have the social and psychological opportunity to surpass with ease the life choices our mothers have made. We come of age, we leave home, and we enter a world in which most social and political institutions have thrown open doors that for thousands of years were closed to women. Therefore, to many of us who have struggled for these very opportunities, it comes as a shock to realize that at that very moment when we might expect to step forward and harvest the fruit of a profound struggle for female liberation, many of the most gifted among us fall prey to a severe suffering that gradually consumes more and more of

our life energy and finally causes what in many cases is a severe breakdown.

(ibid.: 12)

It is in the present generation, then, that women can reap the benefits of feminist struggle for equality with men after 'thousands of years of suppression'; this, then, is a 'historic moment' in which women can for the first time take as their own 'the rights and prerogatives of male society' (ibid.: 19). For Chernin, the present generation of women have been brought up to take equal rights for granted, as a given (ibid.: 28–9).

For Chernin, however, women who suffer from eating disorders – and anorexia in particular – can't say 'yes' to this offered opportunity. She argues that many women feel a 'terror of female development', of taking control of their own lives, and that eating disorders, which occur at times of underlying developmental crisis, regardless of biological age, work subconsciously to prevent movement into the public sphere (ibid.: 21). Life is consumed by the obsession with food – and this obsession is chosen in place of freedom at a turning point in both the individual woman's life and women's history as a whole.

Chernin identifies a number of factors in this collective female refusal of self-development. There is the residue of the historical oppression of women:

> these echoes from history endure; perhaps they have entered so deeply into the fabric of our mind and being that they sound in our ears even today, the silent background to the silent question about the legitimacy of female development.

(ibid.: 32)

Further, women have not traditionally been seen as having the same developmental crises as men, and therefore the culture does not contain rituals with which to express female development (ibid.: 169–70). But far and away the most vital factor in women's failure to take up the promise of development is the mother–daughter relationship.

For Chernin, the new opportunites for women open up historically unprecedented conflicts between mothers and daughters. For the first time, female self-development involves a radical separation from the mother – her values, her way of life, her resignations. The background to this separation, Chernin argues, is a 'progressively growing crisis in the institution of motherhood' (ibid.: 77, 82, 104). In the twentieth century, the concept of the *necessity* of women sacrificing their lives to domesticity, especially motherhood, has broken down under the pressure of women's political struggles. The 'suppositions that were taken for truths' – that women should live through their families, be confined to the domestic sphere and 'give up the longing for their own develop-ment and sacrifice it for their children' – have been gradually broken down (ibid.: 78–9, 125).

Crucially, however, the idea of necessary motherhood has not been replaced with any new theories of womanhood, and without either the belief in domesticity as the inescapable and natural life of woman *or* a viable alternative, the miseries, futilities and discon-tents of domesticity 'break . . . through into consciousness'. The mothers of the post-war era are, then, profoundly discontented. They have only the notion of 'personal fulfillment' to which to refer their lives – and they are inadequate to the challenge (ibid.: 80). *New* assumptions about women's possibilities, such as they are, have come too late for them; unable to accept the necessary sacrifice of their individuality in motherhood, neither can they enter the world of larger possibilities. There is, then, 'a fundamen-tally new type of mother–daughter bond':

> Mothers and daughters of the modern era face one another . . . as beings in a struggle for a self – the older woman having already failed in this quest as the younger starts out on it.
>
> (ibid.: 81)

For the younger woman, then, self-development and self-assertion involve *surpassing* her mother. For the mother, she is ambivalent about her daughter's new opportunities: she wants her daughter to have what she has lacked, but also envies and resents her potential to do so (ibid.: 87–8). Chernin argues:

> there is a marked tendency among women to retreat, to experi-ence a failure of nerve, a debilitating inner conflict about accepting advantages and opportunites denied to their mo-thers. The 'Cinderella complex', the fear of independence from which they are supposedly suffering, is in reality a pervasive worry about our mothers' lives. This anguished concern about the mother is hidden just beneath the surface of the eating problem . . . the contemporary struggle for female identity . . .

in relation to this fateful encounter between a mother whose life has not been fulfilled and a daughter now presented with the opportunity for fulfillment.

(ibid.: 42–3)

It is *guilt*, then, which is at the centre of today's generation of young women's refusal to develop. The daughter is caught between the new images of female power and possibility and the image of 'a fat mother hiding at home', and neither the culture nor her mother can support her (ibid.: 45). The mother, having retreated from self-development herself, cannot support her child through its crises, and the social expectations which allow men to see 'this imperative developmental task, this necessity to face the father at the crossroads and symbolically to kill him and take his place in the world' as a typical and universal 'crisis' do not extend to women (ibid.: 51–3).

For women, then, the idea that 'one generation must proceed inexorably beyond the next' is alien (ibid.: 53, 170). The daughter, faced with the possibility of surpassing her mother in developmental terms, is plagued by guilt, and blames *herself*, rather than her culture, for her mother's wasted life. The daughters feel as though they themselves have 'drained and depleted the mother with the intensity of their needs' (ibid.: 64). Here Chernin draws on the work of Melanie Klein, whose work on the oral-sadistic fantasies of infants suggests that the frustration of the child at its inability to control the food supply leads to destructive impulses towards the mother (ibid.: 117–18; see Klein, 1975). Here, Chernin argues, lie 'the seeds of this hidden mother-rage and mother-guilt which are, at present, restricting our development' (1986: 118). Klein's idea that the child's desire to appropriate the contents first of its mother's breast, then of her whole body, leads to a belief that it has *really* destroyed her is, for Chernin, rather than being a universal truth, dependent on the oppression of women in the institution of motherhood. The belief that, in weaning, the mother has in reality been finally drained dry is bolstered by the more or less simultaneous discovery of the mother's relative *real* powerlessness and depletion by her child's needs. There is, then, a propensity for daughters to feel guilt about their potential to 'surpass' their mothers; the idea that they 'drained' their mothers in reality – an unconscious 'Kleinian memory' – is 'reactivated' in later crises of growth and development (ibid.: 64, 78–93).

Chernin argues:

the terrible guilt we see in a woman with an eating disorder, although it is usually focused on the number of calories consumed and the number of pounds gained, arises from the fact that the woman afflicted with this obsession cannot forgive herself for having damaged her mother in earliest childhood. Consequently, she cannot allow herself to move into the next stages of development, to turn her back on the older woman and leave her behind to the depletion and exhaustion she believes she has inflicted upon her.

(ibid.: 125)

While the son, knowing that he is to become like his father – 'independent, autonomous, involved in the world' – can accept the self-sacrifice of his mother, the daughter, being herself a woman, cannot (ibid.: 126–7). The son is, then, free from guilt, and through 'aggressive fantasies of attack upon the female body' he can also 'manage' *his* 'mother-rage' without attacking himself (ibid.: 129). The daughter, however, is trapped – her anxiety, guilt and anger are *not* culturally transformed, remaining 'stuck' at the level of guilt over food, eating and growth (ibid.: 124, 132–6). Eating remains 'an act of violence against the mother' and this feeling is reinforced by a culture which, Chernin argues, 'fears and dislikes large women' (ibid.: 6). Not eating, then, resolves many guilts – principally, however, the 'primal crime' of imaginary matricide (ibid.: 132).

This, then, is the cause of anorexia:

the daughters of our time are turning against themselves . . . they torture themselves with starvation and make their bodies their enemies . . . they attack their female flesh. This futile attack upon the female body, through which we are attempting to free ourselves from the limitations of the female role, hides a bitter warfare against the mother.

(ibid.: 93)

The guilt and hidden anger at the mother – anger, anxiety and loss at the separation from the mother in weaning – is turned against the female body shared with the mother:

in a stunning act of symbolic substitution, the daughter aims her mother-rage at her own body, so like the one which fed her and

through which she learned to know the mother during the first
moments of her existence.

(ibid.: 93)

She fears that food will turn her into what her mother is –
ambitionless and shameful: 'with every bite she has to fear that she
may become what her mother has been' (ibid.: 42). Anorexia, then,
is an attempt to remake the female body: it is 'symbolic gender
transformation' (ibid.: 52). The daugher hopes that in taking on
the lean, male body, she will 'escape from the mother's destiny
without enduring all that remorse of leaving the mother behind',
and will be able to surpass her mother with the 'serenely cruel and
self-referring' attitude of a son (ibid.: 56). This, however, is impossible – the body regains its natural weight and contours, and
confronts the anorexic woman with 'the fact of being fundamentally and irrevocably female' (ibid.: 53). She is trapped: she can
neither retreat nor go forward.

In eating disorders, then, women transform their bodies because of guilt over transforming their lives and personalities.
Eating disorders should be seen, Chernin argues, as attempts to
evolve 'rites of passage' in which the traditional female identity of
self-sacrificial mother can be transformed and women can enter
the culture. This, she argues, is the purpose of 'tribal' rites of
passage, but because the ritual here is not recognized socially, it is
unable to do this, its 'self-destructive excess' is not controlled, and
ritual thus 'remains split off from its collective significance' (ibid.:
185, 169–86). The anorexic woman 'cannot get beyond these
trappings of transformation' – she remains stuck in the repetition
and elaboration of dietary ritual without experiencing the transformative power of the true rite of passage (ibid.: 175, 174).

This, then, for Chernin, is what is needed: a collective ritual
through which a new female identity can be created – 'intentional
ritual' rather than 'ritualized obsession' (ibid.: 185, 204). She
argues:

> we are in urgent need of a ceremonial form to guide us beyond
> what may well be the collective childhood of female identity into
> a new maturity of female social development.

(ibid.: 169)

Only then will a 'new woman' who can enter the public world
without the finally impossible transformation into a 'pseudo-man'

be born; a woman in whom female creative and nurturing power are integrated in, rather than separated from, her sense of identity.

CRITIQUE OF CHERNIN

Kim Chernin's work is popular, and *The Tyranny of Slenderness* is particularly well known. This is unsurprising – her style is clear, her arguments accessible and her subject relevant to many women. Indeed, Chernin's perspective on anorexia is stimulating and raises many important but often neglected issues – the disjunction between femininity and individuality, the 'problem' of feminine appetites, the opposed orientations of men and women towards the 'public sphere' and the importance of ritual in anorexia.

Especially interesting from my own perspective are her discussions on women's 'inner space', drawn from Melanie Klein. In spite of the fact, as I shall later argue, that I would not accept Chernin's focus on guilt in the mother–daughter relationship as the main explanatory factor in anorexia, the whole area of the imagery of women's bodies as empty inner space is central to the consideration of the body as a *concept* rather than a simple biological given, and will be discussed in later chapters.

However, I would argue that the ahistorical slant of her thesis fundamentally weakens its central arguments. First, arguing that the twentieth century sees the overturning of thousands of years of unmitigated oppression of women is untenable. As Dale Spender, for example, has argued, many of the ideas of contemporary feminism can be traced back as far as the seventeenth century, and Spender charts their emergence, suppression and re-emergence as 'new' (Spender, 1983). It is historically more accurate to see women's struggles against patriarchal oppression as rising and being suppressed, as a struggle both on the material and the ideological levels, and shaped in each period by the specific historical conditions of that time, rather than as one titanic victory over a monolithic and unchanging patriarchy which needs only to be 'rounded off' in the finishing school of female psychology.[1]

I do not wish to suggest that the oppression of women is simply a 'by-product' of capitalism, however. I would argue for the usefulness of the concept of patriarchy, but see it as an overarching concept which should contain within it a wide range of historical differentiation in *how* women are oppressed, and how the oppression of women as a gender intersects with other oppressions, principally those of class and 'race'. Chernin's arguments are based on an extremely simplistic definition of the concept of patriarchy. Her thesis, rather than being informed by history, takes it for granted, and this leads her to vastly underestimate both historical change and the *real* constraints on the expression of female power, arguing that neither the material nor the ideological constraints of patriarchy retain any real effects (Chernin, 1986: 60, 78–80, 90). Thus Chernin downgrades women's continuing economic, ideological and political subordination and only gives glancing consideration to the patriarchal control of the female body which must be central to any feminist analysis of anorexia (ibid.: 115). This, for a feminist, is a staggering feat of non-recognition. As Janet Sayers argues, in order to end women's oppression we need more than a new attitude to mother–daughter relationships:

> we have to do more than 'dream of the future, out of the transformed obsessions that presently rule our lives' as Chernin recommends [ibid.: 204]. We also have to take practical steps to actualise this dream in reality . . . Sadly Chernin . . . fails adequately to detail the means whereby the solution she advocates to sex inequality might be realised in practice.
>
> (Sayers: 1987)

In line with her theory that equality for women has been wholly achieved for the present generation, Chernin sees the social controls on women which continue to keep femininity and domesticity on the female agenda as mere 'echoes from history' (1986: 32), and as relating solely to patriarchy. This latter strand in her argument is best seen in her treatment of middle-class women as representative of *all* women, the issues of their specific class *and* gender position as issues affecting all women equally. Indeed it is the very fact that young, educated, white Western women are in a *specialized* position both in terms of gender, 'race' and class that access to the public/male sphere has become an issue for *them*.

Women, for Chernin, then, seem to be a largely self-oppressing group – the constraints which keep women from moving fully into the public sphere exist primarily in the minds of women themselves and apply equally to all women, regardless of their class position or ethnic background. There is a glancing recognition that women may not be doing it all to themselves when Chernin writes of the anorexic woman's 'brooding, half-conscious sense that her culture, after opening the doors to its most highly prized

institutions, does not really welcome female development at all'
(ibid.: 187). This point, unfortunately, remains unexplored, as
does the question of whether the culture opens its doors wider for
some women than for others. Guilt is seen as a purely internal and
irrational mechanism, not as an element in the *social* control of
women through which women 'police' themselves.

The 'failure of nerve' is women's, the conflicts psychological
(ibid.: 43). To take one example, Chernin argues that there is a
'battle of opposing imagery' between 'the new image of female
possibility' and the traditional image of mother-in-the-kitchen,
and that it is women's 'guilt' at surpassing their mothers which
prevents them from embracing the new possibilities (ibid.: 45).
This perspective totally ignores the profound ambiguity in images
of powerful women, informed by stereotypes of the wicked step-
mother – women's power is bad power – or the pseudo-man –
powerful women are unfeminine. The attitudes of *both* genders
towards women who 'make it' in a man's world are highly ambiguous.

It is here that the central confusion in Chernin's argument
begins to show itself. She argues that women often feel the lack of
a 'self', that women do not have the expectation of surpassing and
therefore fully separating from their mothers in the way that men
do, and that there is a basic conflict between femininity – sublimat-
ing the self to live through others – and individualism – acting as
a separate and autonomous person (ibid.: 20, 125–9). In spite of
her caveats on the need to take into account woman-as-nurturer
– this latter also presented as a universal and ahistorical quality –
the model of the self from which she works more or less uncritically
is the atomized and self-contained individual of bourgeois and
patriarchal ideology.

Chernin does, as we have seen, argue that women cannot, or
should not, attempt to solve their problems by becoming 'pseudo-
men' – here coming close to arguing that the dominant concepts
of the self do not 'fit' women's experience. However, this does not
lead her to question the naturalness and universality of the
atomized self which struggles to separate from and supersede the
parent. This struggle is, for Chernin, expressive of 'basic psychological needs' and is thus an 'inevitable', 'human necessity' (ibid.:
169–70). Indeed, in her discussion of pre-modern 'tribal' rites of
passage she argues that separation/individuation has always been
their main function (ibid.: 166–71). Here, I would argue, she

ignores the fundamental distinction, to be discussed in later chapters, between the pre-modern definition of the self by social role and the modern self as defined by individualized 'personality'.

Women's present position is described as 'the collective childhood of female identity' (ibid.: 169), and we can have little doubt about what 'a new maturity' would mean. Although some traits – aggression, for example – are seen to be male, and others – nurturing, creativity – female, Chernin retains the sense of the self acting upon an environment from which it is totally separated as gender-neutral, and as something 'authentic' which can be discovered, rather than as a social, and therefore historical, *construction* (ibid.: 195–200).

As I shall argue later in more depth, a wholehearted commitment to the social construction of personality negates the need to posit a 'natural' or 'authentic' – in Chernin's terms – self which exists independently of culture, history and the gender division. I would argue that the dominant conception of the self as a self-contained entity organized around a core of needs/desires which are satisfied through the exploitation of an environment composed of objects is masculine and bourgeois, rather than gender-neutral and universal. Further, this construction relies upon, and is constructed in opposition to, a conception of woman as fundamentally 'un-separate', as, indeed, part of the environment of objects through which the masculine subject expresses itself.

The institution of motherhood, then, is *one* expression of the 'lack of self' which women experience in the collision of bourgeois individualism and patriarchal femininity. The mother lives through her children because responsiveness to the needs and desires of others is central to patriarchal definitions of feminine personality, but even the childless woman cannot achieve the masculine self. Self-effacement is not solely the province of mothers, and guilt is not produced solely in the mother–daughter relationship. It is not women who confine themselves to the manipulation of the body, fearing to 'take on' the public world. Rather, patriarchal power confines them.

In essence, then, Chernin psychologizes and domesticates a social and political conflict – the control of women through patriarchal power realtions. Women's search for 'identity' is stifled in a purely domestic psychodrama which 'culture' merely 'reinforces' from the 'outside', there being in Chernin's thesis no *real* struggle

to retain culture as patriarchal. The struggle is seen as psychological and domestic, rather than social, material and ideological,
between the formal gender-neutrality of the concept of the individual and the patriarchal control of women through the ideology
of femininity.

I would argue, in short, that Chernin's analysis of anorexia can
only hold water if we accept that the patriarchal oppression of
women is effectively over, and that the 'masculine' self is the proper
goal of women. If we do not, we will be forced to look outside of
the mother–daughter relationship to the wider social forces which
continue to oppress and constrain women – as mothers and
daughters certainly, but also as wives, girlfriends, workers and
citizens. If we do so we liberate the analysis of anorexia from its
dependence on a particular 'type' of mother – the discontented
woman ambivalent about her daughter's growth – and the control
of feminine appetite can be understood as social rather than
self-inflicted.

MARILYN LAWRENCE: CONTROL AND CONTAINMENT

Marilyn Lawrence is the most widely read feminist writer on
anorexia; her book *The Anorexic Experience* (1984a) is frequently
cited, and she has done extensive therapeutic work with anorexic
women.

For Lawrence, anorexia is a strategy of control which operates
at two levels. First, at the physical level, the anorexic woman tries
through her eating and non-eating strategies to gain and maintain
complete control over the size and shape of her body. Second, at
the moral level, the anorexic woman tries to gain and maintain
control over her needs and desires through strategies of self-
denial. These attempts to achieve 'perfect and absolute control'
are motivated by a feeling of being *out* of control, which also occurs
at two levels: physically, as expressed in the fear of becoming fat;
and morally, in seeing themselves as 'glutinous and debased'
(Lawrence, 1979: 93).

Anorexic women, Lawrence argues, want to control what happens in their lives, a control which women's relative social
powerlessness problematizes. The reality of this powerlessness
means that it is very difficult for women to exert a controlling
influence over their actual social position (ibid.: 93, 100). Self-
control through control of the body *is* possible, however, and it is

this turning inward of the attempt at control which anorexia effects:

> In order for an individual to be free to direct herself and take charge of her own actions, it is necessary for her to engage with other people in such a way that the interaction allows her this control. It may be necessary for her to exercise some power in relation to other people. When anorexics talk about control, they invariably mean the power to regulate, command and govern their own lives and actions. They generally fail to do this by turning outwards and engaging with the world on their own behalf. Instead, they exercise self-control, which we might understand as power turned inwards. The battleground then becomes an internal one: the battle is fought within the individual rather than between the individual and the world.
>
> (ibid.: 93)

Anorexic women experience women's relative social powerlessness as 'a total inability to control the environment', and 'compensate' for this with rigid self-control (ibid.: 94). This control of the self works through a sharp definition of *boundaries*:

> Anorexics appear to need to separate themselves from the environment. They need to define their own limits and set boundaries around themselves. The setting of boundaries around the self is a difficult problem for women as they are at least in part regarded as an aspect of the environment of others . . . Being very thin seems to say to the world 'I have sharp contours, I am not soft, I do not merge with you. I have nothing to give you.' A recovered anorexic vividly described her anorexic experience . . . in terms of 'needing to be closed up for a while, and very small. Not receptive, not there for others.'
>
> (ibid.: 94)

Lawrence argues that anorexic physical self-control should be divided analytically into a control of weight and shape, and a control of intake, with the former functioning as 'tangible proof' that the latter is working (ibid.: 95). Self-denial, then, expressed in the rigorous control of appetite, is central to anorexia: 'Anorexia is an attempt to deny appetite, to rise above appetite and everything which appetite implies' (1984a: 89; see also Lawrence, 1987: 195). The anorexic woman fears that 'her own feelings, needs and

longings will be too much for herself and for other people to bear'
(1984a: 100).

Anorexia is, then, a kind of asceticism (1979: 94; 1984a: 33).
Lawrence argues that in our culture self-denial is regarded as a
'"good" thing' for everyone, but especially for women, who are
'more inherently prone to badness and moral weakness' (1979: 95;
1984a: 18, 33–5). Anorexic women use 'almost precisely' the
methods of medieval female ascetics 'to achieve the same ends'
(1979: 96).

The reasons why the search for control and denial is instigated
through control of eating and the body are to be found in an
examination of the subordinate social position of women. First,
food and eating are major female concerns, and anorexia can be
viewed as an extension of the difficulties *all* women have with
eating:

> it [anorexia] is in fact at one end of a continuum of confused and
> conflicted responses which we as women have towards our-
> selves . . . we do not just eat: we slim, we worry, we weight
> watch. We also spend an inordinate amount of time absorbed
> in the business of food: feeding others as well or instead of
> ourselves, shopping, cooking, and clearing-up the waste . . .
> Food in our society . . . is regarded as the responsibility of
> women. It is one of the few areas of life in which we are expected
> to be in control.
>
> (1984a, 12, 18, 28; see also 1987: 12)

Second, the control and manipulation of the body is also a major
facet of female existence. Lawrence argues that appearance is
central to women's acceptability, and today sexual acceptability
demands slimness (1984a: 33–42). Weight control, therefore, is
commonplace in women's lives, both in the attempt to conform to
a cultural stereotype, and as an expression of the idea that if
women experience problems, they should change themselves
rather than their society in order to deal with them (1979: 94;
1984a: 21). Control of food and the body is accessible to women,
and because of the relative powerlessness inherent in women's
subordinate position in society, food and the body are two of the
few areas open to female control (1979: 100).

The attempt to control eating and the body is, then, for Lawrence a method or strategy of control, chosen partly for its existing
place in the culture of femininity and partly through lack of

alternatives. But it is merely the *method*. Although 'the key feature of anorexia is an unshakeable desire to control both food intake and weight' (1979: 94), for Lawrence, following Bruch: 'in spite of outer appearances, this is not an illness of weight and appetite – the essential problem relates to inner doubts and lack of self-confidence' (1984: 77). The underlying conflict of anorexia, then – its *real* cause – is for Lawrence, as for Bruch, a conflict over independence and autonomy (1979: 97). At adolescence 'issues about autonomy, independence and self-esteem . . . come to a head' (1984a: 49). The anorexic girl, having always accepted the valued female qualities of compliance, passivity and unselfishness, has seen herself through others' definitions and lacks a clear sense of self. Thus: 'when she reaches the point in her life at which independence and autonomy are required, she is likely to feel unable to cope' (ibid.: 65). She can neither achieve nor maintain 'a sense of herself as a free and autonomous person' (ibid.: 66).

Crucial in this crisis are the educational pressures which the usually middle-class anorexic girl faces, where pressure to do well academically and subsequently in a career conflicts with the social pressures on women to be carers, 'to find satisfaction through affiliation' (ibid.: 53; 1979: 201–5).[2] The conflict, then, is between two courses of action: pursuing individualistic success which is seen to involve a *rejection* of affiliation and femininity; or abandoning this course to become fully feminine and therefore subordinate, defining the self in relation to the needs of others (1979: 204–5).

Anorexia is a way to step outside this conflict, and should be seen as 'a retreat from independence' (1984a: 67). The conflict is social rather than individual as, for Lawrence, it is not the anorexic girl herself who is confused due to her *own* inadequacies, but rather the social world which is riven with conflicts over how adult women should behave (ibid.: 74). Anorexia is thus 'a disorder which springs from the very midst of women's experience of the world' (ibid.: 21). In summary, then:

> One of the central elements in anorexia is the tendency to want to please and to comply with other people's expectations. It is when complying and pleasing others becomes incompatible with the demands of real maturity and autonomy that anorexia tends to occur. It is the failure to take into account the real needs of the self and to clearly differentiate these from the needs of

others which heralds the onset of the rebellious symptom in the first place.

(ibid.: 85)

The anorexic girl, then, tries to impose control – in the only way that she perceives to be possible – in response to conflicts and confusions which appear insoluble. Lawrence distinguishes the *aim* of anorexia – in which the anorexic girl tries to retreat from confusion and conflicts between 'success' (primarily educational) and dependent femininity – and the *method* used to achieve this aim, which she describes as the attempt, through physical and moral control strategies, to construct a 'shell' around the self:

> we can think of the symptoms of anorexia as a kind of protective outer shell. The shell is not the real person, but it hides and protects the real person. The important point is that the real self is still there, underneath . . . using her anorexia ['Stella'] . . . created an outer shell which was strong and invulnerable. It did not need love, it did not need friendship, it did not need food. It had no connection with anyone or anything in its environment. It was complete and contained within itself. It had declared its independence.

(ibid.: 22–3)

Anorexia means living 'within and behind the walls of your solution'; it is 'in a real sense a "No Entry" sign' (ibid.: 21): 'the goal is self-sufficiency, the achievement of a steady state within a closed system. Nothing can change. Nothing must enter' (ibid.: 202). The anorexic solution, however, cannot be permanent or total. Most anorexic women eat at least something. The body can never come *absolutely* under moral control, and the anorexic woman lives with the constant need to increase control by decreasing intake. Lawrence argues thus: 'the road to self-respect through starvation is an endless one, because the goal doesn't really lie in that direction' (1979: 98).

The anorexic woman is also terrified that her appetite will overwhelm her and that she will eat uncontrollably (ibid.: 97–9) and feels as though she is 'in a state of siege' (1984a: 19). Further, the anorexic process itself 'gets out of hand', and instead of the woman herself controlling her eating, *it* seems to control her. One of Lawrence's clients described this feeling thus: 'My willpower is stronger than I am' (1979: 100). Lawrence writes:

what brings anorexics to therapy (and by this I mean a voluntary asking for help) is the conviction that they are out of control. Universally they claim that they cannot control what is happening to them, whether this be over-eating, under-eating or a combination of the two. I have two clients (both of a religious disposition) who firmly believed that they were in the grip of some evil demon which tormented them whenever they attempted to eat.

(ibid.: 98)

The anorexic strategy, put simply, does not work:

it is a solution which is symptomatic of the desperate situation it seeks to rectify. It is a solution which is essentially self-destructive and which seeks to substitute self-control for effective control of the world in which the woman exists.

(ibid.: 100)

CRITIQUE OF LAWRENCE

In going on to discuss and criticize Marilyn Lawrence's work on anorexia, I would like again to distinguish this critique from my earlier critique of psychiatric definitions of anorexia. The latter, as has been shown, base their explanations of anorexia on individualist and phallocentric assumptions, arguing that anorexia is both explicable and curable at the individual level, and that the concept of the healthy, mature and psychologically 'normal' adult is gender-neutral. I have argued that these assumptions are essentially *ideological*, and this point will be explored further in later chapters.

Feminist theories of anorexia, however, are developed from a position which is potentially critical of these assumptions. First, feminists seek explanations of anorexia not in the concept of the deficient individual, but in the social position of women as a group, arguing here, as elsewhere, that the personal is political. Second, much feminist work on gender roles argues that they are social constructions rather than eternal, biologically determined realities.[3] From both a sociological and a feminist perspective, therefore, my work shares the feminist critique of patriarchal ideology, and what I hope to do here is *deepen* and *develop*, rather than undermine or reject, the feminist theories I have chosen to focus on.

To return to Marilyn Lawrence's work, it should be clear that from a feminist and sociological perspective her analysis of anorexia represents a major theoretical advance. In seeing anorexia as a product of the social position of women, in pointing out the importance of food and appearance in the female gender role, in questioning how far 'independence' is a real possibility for women, and in arguing for a connection between the anorexic strategy and women's relative social powerlessness, Lawrence provides an effective explanation of anorexia as a *female* condition. After reading Lawrence we can see clearly, and for the first time, why the anorexic experience is meaningful almost exclusively to women.

I would, however, argue that Lawrence's work contains some conceptual confusions, and also that the therapeutic focus of some of her work can lead to a critical lack of depth in her analysis. Although she explicitly argues for an explanation of anorexia grounded in analysis of the social position of women, this analysis remains largely undeveloped, specifically in its historical aspect. The feminist theoretical framework must be much more fully understood, I would argue, if we are to use such concepts as 'independence', 'dependence', and 'powerlessness' in explaining anorexia.

Further, there is a crucial ambiguity in Lawrence's acceptance of the social genesis of anorexia. In *The Anorexic Experience* she seems to suggest that, although it is understandable socially, anorexia is, to some degree at least, also explicable by individual psychological deficiency, the anorexic girl being unable to resolve social confusions in any more productive way, not having 'found a way of being in the world which is both comfortable and realistic' (1984a: 55). The implication here, then, is that conflicting *social* expectations of women – to 'succeed' as individuals and to subordinate themselves to the needs of others – can indeed be reconciled at the *individual* level. What is needed for women who have been unable to resolve these conflicts themselves is therapy which will set them on the way to that resolution which, we must assume, other women have already achieved (1979: 100). It should of course be noted that Lawrence does identify critically one other 'resolution' of this conflict – giving up on individual success to concentrate on femininity (1984a: 54).

Two points arise here. First, as Lawrence argues (1979), anorexia *is* an attempt, however unproductive, to resolve conflicting expectations central in the lives of middle-class women. This view fits ill with her later argument that anorexia represents a 'retreat' from conflicts over independence, a 'regression' into dependence (1984a: 67). Further, I see anorexia as one 'resolution' among many, and would argue that is important not to set up, albeit implicitly, a distinction between women along lines of their relative success in dealing with cultural expectations which, in varying degrees and in various ways, oppress us all as 'members' of the gender-group 'woman'.

Second, I would question the extent to which individual therapeutic solutions can engage with anorexia as a *social* phenomenon. While therapy which takes seriously the political issues involved in anorexia, and allows the anorexic woman to retain control of her life, can be very effective, it treats the 'effects' rather than the 'cause'. Therapy can help women as individuals come to terms with the reality of social powerlessness in hopefully less painful ways, but it does not attack the social structure which produces that powerlessness in the first place. If we accept the analysis of anorexia as arising from women's position in the social structure, we must surely accept that therapy can help women who are already anorexic but cannot prevent other women becoming anorexic in the future.

I also find somewhat problematic Lawrence's displacement of the anorexic *method* – control of eating – from the heart of her analysis. While I accept that a dependence/independence conflict lies at the heart of anorexia I would argue that anorexic eating should be seen not simply as a 'method' chosen because of its place in the lives of women to achieve a distinct 'aim'. *Why* and *how* this specific 'method' expresses the conflict between individuality and femininity are questions which will be central in later chapters. The relationship of 'method' and 'aim', I would argue, needs to be rigorously theorized. There are good reasons for the control of eating being 'chosen' to express conflicts over dependence, reasons which I shall explore in later chapters. My argument, briefly, is that the active pursuit of self-interest and the satisfaction of desire are central facets of the bourgeois construction of the individual. In patriarchal ideology and practice, however, women are constructed as the passive objects of the desires of the masculine subject, rather than the active pursuers of their own desires. Feminine desire, feminine behaviour, is constructed as *responsive* to masculine action, as dependent upon it. Independent, unresponsive desire is expected of individuals but sanctioned in women, through, for example, the construction of autonomous female desire as dangerous, voracious and potentially overwhelming. It is much more than lack of confidence which prevents women controlling their own destinies. Thus independence and appetite, dependence and denial are inextricably linked. Indeed, it is the expression of these links in anorexia which excites sociological interest.

To return to Lawrence, what I am suggesting of her analysis is, then, that while it links self-denial and gender it apprehends but fails to adequately theorize the links between individuality, desire and gender in a specifically *bourgeois* culture, the links between who we are, what we want, and what we can have. The issue of appetite in anorexia which Lawrence so interestingly raises in her earlier work remains unfortunately undeveloped in later writings.

We need to look at feminine appetite, then, as it is understood in bourgeois and patriarchal culture. The attempt to establish boundaries around the self, too, would benefit from a similar treatment. The notion of the individual as a coherent and self-contained unit is both historically and gender-specific, and is reflected in the social construction of the body. The pseudo gender-neutral ideology of individualism presents the goals of self-contained selfhood and bodily integrity for women as possible, while simultaneously the ideology of femininity creates the feminine self *in response to* the masculine self, the feminine body in relation to the masculine body, and thus continually undercuts any real possibility that women will achieve those goals.

The feminine body in bourgeois and patriarchal culture is understood, I will later argue, as incomplete. Lawrence's argument that anorexia represents the construction of a psychic 'shell' or boundary is thus a vital component in the development of theoretical connections between the cultural meanings of the female body and the anorexic experience, and I am indebted to her for this element of my argument. I would suggest, however, that Lawrence does not sufficiently detail either how the anorexic 'shell' is constructed or how the social construction of the feminine body as open makes it meaningful.

This level of argument, however, requires a specifically *sociological* perspective on personality development and on the body. From this point of view 'personality', or 'human nature', and the body are seen as social constructions rather than as universal givens, and thus incorporate the social divisions and categorizations of their

era. To the extent that definitions of 'personality' lack this perspective such definitions are essentialist, in presenting the
individualized self as universal, and phallocentric, in presenting
the masculine self as gender-neutral.

I would argue that in spite of her feminist perspective Lawrence
falls at least partly into the traps of phallocentrism and essential-
ism. Her description of the goal of treatment in anorexia seems to
implicitly accept the individualized self as the model on which her
patients should focus, an acceptance which seems to contain little
recognition of either its historical or its gender-specificity.

There is confusion in her work between the idea that the
anorexic woman has no sense of self at all, and the idea that her
'real self' is still there 'underneath'. Further, the conflicts between
'compliance' and 'responsiveness' as gender-role requirements for
women and the need for the patient to act according to 'the real
needs of the self', 'the demands of real maturity and autonomy'
(1984a: 85; see also 1987: 203) are not theoretically resolved. Thus,
the ideological interface of femininity and individualism is never
directly addressed by Lawrence: we are shown its effects – i.e. in
education (Lawrence, 1984b) – but must construe its nature and
extent for ourselves.

There is, then, an underlying ambiguity in Lawrence's view of
individuality. Although her feminism leads her to criticize the
effects of the female gender-role on personality, she continues to
maintain that a 'real' self exists independently of such effects – and,
indeed, independently of *any* aspect of social structure. This allows
her to argue that recognizing the 'real self' and its needs will solve
the anorexic crisis of independence; unfortunately, it also allows
her to ignore the extent to which self-contained individuality is a
real possibility for women. Lawrence's long-term therapeutic aim
is to enable the anorexic woman 'to take a proper and reasonable
control of her own life . . .[and] to become an effective agent in her
own affairs' (1984a: 81), to encourage her to see that she 'owns'
her own body (ibid.: 93) and that she can act 'according to internal
rather than external demands' (1987: 203). She seems to suggest
that women can simply 'decide' to be autonomous individuals
rather than dependent accessories, since this is what they 'really
are' underneath. I would argue, however, that the conflicts between 'individuality' and the constraints of the feminine
gender-role are not soluble simply by adopting a different perspec-

tive, or by therapy (even feminist therapy) but require social change.

At some level Lawrence does recognize this point, arguing that anorexia: 'is really an attempt to hold together an identity, and to avoid the loss of one part of the self which growing up brings with it' (1984b: 206). Here she argues that in pre-puberty a girl can be *both* 'pretty' – that is, an acceptable female – *and* 'clever' – a successful individual. At puberty, however, she has to choose: she hits 'the friction-point of womanhood' (ibid.: 204). Although in her article on education (1984b) Lawrence implicitly presents 'identity' itself as a social construction, elsewhere she seems to see it as universal, existing a priori, 'under' the effects of the gender division. The assumption here seems to be that 'underneath' the gender division we are all really the same, and would remain so were it not that different 'tendencies' are 'encouraged' in women and men (1984a: 49, 53).

The ahistoricism of Lawrence's analysis is also evident in the way she uses the concept of asceticism. Lawrence 'lifts' the concept out of feudal culture and argues that anorexic women in contemporary culture use the same ascetic methods in pursuit of the same aims as did medieval female ascetics. In Chapter 1 I argued that this use of the term by Bell was unsound, and the same criticisms apply here.

I would argue, then, that Lawrence's concept of 'selfhood' remains somewhat confused, and that this stems both from a commitment to therapy over analysis and from a too uncritical acceptance of psychiatric definitions of the normal individual and the bourgeois and patriarchal ideology which creates those definitions. In spite of this confusion, however, Lawrence's definition of anorexia as a strategy of control, arising from a conflict between independence and femininity, pursued through the creation of a psychic 'shell' is, I would argue, the most accurate and comprehensive analysis to be found in the literature.

SUSIE ORBACH: MOTHERS AND DAUGHTERS 2

Susie Orbach's interest in anorexia is pre-dated by her work, both theoretical and practical, on 'compulsive eating' in particular, and female psychology in general. *Fat is a Feminist Issue*, a bestseller, argues that women use body-size to express feelings which are otherwise inexpressible (Orbach, 1978). With Luise Eichenbaum, she isolates neediness and dependency as central issues in the psychology of women (Orbach and Eichenbaum, 1983). Both aspects of her earlier work can be seen in her analysis of anorexia.

In *Hunger Strike*, Orbach argues that anorexia consists of two processes: the pursuit of thinness, and the denial of emotional neediness (Orbach, 1986). The anorexic woman is engaged in a transformation of her body, the aim of which is thinness, but during the illness the meaning of the symptom changes, and its goal becomes the control of eating and the body, rather than simple thinness. It is losing control which comes to terrify the anorexic, and Orbach argues that denial of food and bodily control are symbolic of the denial and control of *emotional* needs (ibid.: 13–14). The anorexic woman 'speaks with her body':

> Her body is a statement about her and the world and her statement about her position in the world. Living within prescribed boundaries, women's bodies become the vehicle for a whole range of expressions that have no other medium. The body, offered as a woman's ticket into society . . . becomes her mouthpiece. In her attempts to conform to or reject contemporary ideals of femininity, she uses the weapon so often directed against her. She speaks with her body.
>
> (ibid.: 48)

Anorexia, then, is a language and a protest: it expresses unconsciously a 'solution' to problems which cannot be consciously articulated (ibid.: 17).

Orbach identifies three factors in the changing role of women in Western society which determine the formation of the anorexic symptom. In consumer society, she argues, women's bodies are 'the ultimate commodity', and are, to women and to men, 'objects of alienation, fascination and desire' (ibid.: 35; 37). Women's bodies and women's sexuality are seen 'from the outside' as objects, and this has two effects. First, the manipulation of the body-as-object in order to make it acceptable is a constant reality for women; and second, women cannot have 'an unmediated or purely physical relation to their bodies' (ibid.: 36). Both manipulation of the body-as-object and a 'mediated' relationship to the body are expressed in anorexia.

The second factor is the post-Second World War confusion over motherhood, where the concept of biologically destined motherhood was challenged by women's increasing dissatisfaction with domesticity and their search for a life outside the home (ibid.: 37–42). Orbach argues that for the mothers and daughters of this time confusion and uncertainty about what a woman should be and how mothers should behave was endemic; anorexia, then, in its rigid control of the body 'is a symbolic attempt to forge a consistency where little exists, to provide a knowable, reliable way of being that can withstand the demand for change' (ibid.: 42).

Finally, and relatedly, the mother–daughter relationship is itself necessarily ambivalent. The mother has to bring up her daughter to accept an inferior social position, to subsume her needs in the needs of others and to live a 'circumscribed life', while at the same time wanting the best for her (ibid.: 43). Anorexia is one way in which the daughter can express the ambivalent relationship to physical and emotional needs which she has learned from her mother.

Needs, for Orbach, are central both in anorexia and in the development of a self. It is the development of a core of needs and desires, both emotional and physical, experienced as existing within the self which creates the individual as separate. The knowledge that what you feel inside, what you want and need, is acceptable and can be consistently met and validated by the world outside your self/body is what gives the individual the sense of him/herself as a separate, self-contained entity, that is, 'a corporeal sense of self', the sense of being 'a physical/mental unit' (ibid.: 77; 76–88). Orbach argues:

> the development of a corporeal sense of self is entirely related to the development of object relations (relations to others beginning with the recognition of the mother as a person, an object separate from oneself).
>
> (ibid.: 77)

> The capacity to experience oneself as a separate person, as a subject (to individuate) rests on the gratification of early dependency needs.
>
> (ibid.: 45–6)

The security that these needs can be satisfied readily is central to a sense of self; women do not have their early needs satisfied consistently and thus their sense of self is shaky (ibid.: 18). This inconsistency operates both emotionally and physically – girls are fed less and weaned earlier – and creates confusion about the acceptability of emotional and physical needs. Because her mother did not respond consistently to her 'internal cues', the daughter experiences them as insatiable. Her ego does not 'integrate' around her needs, and there is thus no 'internal sense of continuity and security' around which the self can develop (ibid.: 81, 108–9, 46, 54, 91). The girl's self thus remains 'embryonic' (ibid.: 109).

Orbach identifies three 'basic demands' of femininity which undermine this self-development: women must defer to others, anticipate and meet others' needs, and seek self-definition through connection with another. Being successfully feminine results in 'a shaky sense of self', where women 'are unable to develop an authentic sense of their needs or a feeling of entitlement for their desires' (ibid.: 43). Women take care of others' needs and respond to others' desires but are fundamentally unsure and ashamed of their *own* desires, and thus find 'psychosomatic unity' difficult to achieve (ibid.: 104). Paradoxically, however, women must appear dependent, and thus their own needs 'thwarted and unmet, go underground' (ibid.: 44). The mother transmits and the daughter receives the idea that women's needs are often unacceptable, the mother failing actively to encourage the daughter's initiatives or adequately and consistently to meet her early needs. Thus, initiating action and satisfying desire remains fraught with difficulty for women, as does psychological separation (ibid.: 45). Women 'deny, ignore or suppress many needs and initiatives that arise internally' and because of this 'grow up with a sense of never having received quite enough, and often feel insatiable and unfulfilled' (ibid.: 78).

When issues of separation and individuation are 're-evoked' in adolescence, then, 'the struggle for an identity separate from the family is made on fairly shaky foundations' (ibid.: 46). The fact that in puberty her body changes in ways she cannot control 'rock[s] the young woman's already tenuous psychic foundations' (ibid.: 47) and her insecurity with her self beomes transposed into an insecurity with the body, exacerbated by her mother's inability to convey unambigously the 'positive aspects of female sexuality' (ibid.: 79). She seeks the external reassurance and control of dieting, and resolves the issue of unacceptable neediness through a rigid control of hunger, a transformation for which her early problems with eating had already prepared her. She denies and controls her need for food as a metaphor for her denial and control of a needy self (ibid.: 48). Her aim is to 'disassociate herself from her body, to not be in her body or to exist as a non-corporeal being'.

The embryonic needy self/body is rejected, and a 'false' self/body devoid of needs is projected (ibid.:89). Orbach, following Winnicott, explains:

> The self that one has put forward in the expression of need is implicitly rejected by the caretaker in her failure to respond appropriately to those needs. The psyche then protectively develops a more pleasing 'false self' ... devoid of the needs and the initiations which seemed to push the much-needed caretaker away.
>
> (ibid.: 89)

This concept is extended to include a 'false body':

> where the developing child has not had a chance to experience its physicality as good, wholesome and essentially all right, it has little chance to live in an authentically experienced body. A false body is then fashioned which conceals the feelings of discomfort and insecurity with regard to the hidden or undeveloped 'inner body'.
>
> (ibid.: 89)

Orbach argues, like Palazzoli, that the body, in object-relations terms, comes to represent the negative aspects of the mother-as-object, the aspects that could not meet the child's needs, as well as the 'bad' needs themselves. The anorexic woman's alienation from her body represents her alienation from both the bad object and her needs. But although she rejects her body, it is at the same time 'all that she has' (ibid.: 90).

The 'unnurtured real self ...[is] split off and repressed' and the anorexic woman withdraws from the disappointing outer environment (ibid.: 89–90). The body 'has come to represent the existence and insistence of needs', and the emaciated anorexic body is 'the tangible evidence . . . that she has indeed done away with the unacceptable self' (ibid.: 151).

Anorexia, then, is an attempt to form a boundary around the self through the control of eating and the body as a substitute for the boundary around the 'stable core' of internal needs, which would 'arise spontaneously as a result of a smooth journey through the process of separation/individuation' (ibid.: 176) if those needs were consistently met, as they are for the non-anorexic child, whose needs, having been 'correctly interpreted in early childhood' can be met as an adult 'without undue difficulty' (ibid.: 91).

Anorexia is a 'somatized solution' to the feelings of uncontrollable and chaotic neediness, 'a much needed defence against the exposure of a very vulnerable nascent "me"' (ibid.: 91).

During the illness, however, the *conscious* denial of food is transformed, and food refusal becomes involuntary (ibid.: 97). Eating becomes a dangerous and 'illegitimate' activity, food 'a forbidden substance' to which the anorexic woman has no right (ibid.: 99). Orbach explains:

> For the anorectic woman there is both an active and a passive relationship to food. This is a complex idea. An originally *active* desire or decision not to eat or to reduce one's food intake soon melds into an experience in which the anorexic feels herself *unable* to eat . . . the rituals and regulations that come to circumscribe her food intake tend to increase in number, gradually taking on a life of their own in such a way that it becomes impossible for her to envision eating in a spontaneous way. Thus the original act of deciding consciously to intervene to reduce her eating becomes not so much a moment to moment act of refusal but rather the consequence of the labyrinth of restrictive practices that in effect prevent her from eating.
>
> (ibid.: 100–1)

The denial is never enough, and it is never over; its original purpose of thinness and acceptability is overtaken by the struggle not to lose control (ibid.: 107). Anorexia, then, is 'only tangentially about slimness', the real function of which is to prove that denial is working (ibid.: 109–10).

The anorexic girl hears the same social messages about the unacceptability of female desire as do all women, but she hears them 'in quadrophonic sound' (ibid.: 114). The individual's experience, Orbach argues, has 'social roots', and the psychoanalytic account of the inner world of the anorexic woman must be read in the context of the sociological account of the position of all women, in which women are food-providers but are at the same time expected to deny themselves food in order to maintain a stereotypical body-image (ibid.: 66–76). The anorexic 'solution' depends on the central importance of body-image in women's experience; without this anorexia would not be 'an appropriate response and protest' (ibid.: 66). Orbach argues that a woman's identity is dependent on her body, and that women's subjective experience of their bodies is mediated by 'cultural factors outside themselves', by a 'social overlay' of meanings and images (ibid.: 70). In this thinness is crucial, and she argues that the emergence of thinness as an ideal for women precisely at the time when women, in the second wave of public feminism, were demanding more public space, is no coincidence (ibid.: 75). Bodily insecurity, then, is a reality for all women.

Further, Orbach argues that in our culture, because of female nurturing, 'the power of the mother is deeply embedded in each of our psychologies' (ibid.: 82). She uses Dinnerstein's argument that men 'reject the power of the mother through the political and psychological subjugation of women' to explain 'the cultural propensity to control women's bodies' (ibid.: 83). The desire to control the mother denied to 'the omnipotent infantile part of the personality' is 'somewhat assuaged' by the control of women's bodies and female sexuality (ibid.: 84–5).

Both at the psychological and the social level, therefore, what is needed is an acceptance of female desire as legitimate. The personal solution to body-image problems must go hand in hand with the extension of the scope of women's lives and the transformation of patriarchal social relations and the images of women they produce (ibid.: 192). The anorexic woman must be helped, through therapy, to develop a 'psychological and corporeal sense of self in which needs for contact, needs for hunger and other physical appetites could be acknowledged' and the acceptability of their satisfaction established (ibid.: 91, 134, 165). The therapist's aim is to show that desire and its implementation are not in themselves essentially fearful or negative, to provide an environment of 'emotional reliability' in which needs get addressed and are thus seen as acceptable (ibid.: 170, 141). The anorexic woman will thus develop her embryonic self to a level at which she can satisfy her needs in a self-regulated way, and achieve psychosomatic unity – the experience of the body as owned and lived in (ibid.: 145–53). She can then speak directly, rather than through her body.

Orbach concludes:

The corrective emotional food then makes it possible for her to approach the wider environment differently as a potential source of self-expression and nurture. In allowing herself to feel and to act she reverses some of the key features of socialization towards femininity . . . she becomes a person with legitimate desires and demands which she can now openly express.

(ibid.: 179–80)

CRITIQUE OF ORBACH

Hunger Strike is an immensely valuable book. Susie Orbach's analysis is thoughtful, compassionate and helpful. Especially valuable is her focus on the issue of 'needs' in anorexia: locating anorexia as an aspect of the social control of female desire is a huge step forward from the individual pathology standpoint of psychiatric ideology. The notions of anorexia as an attempt to create boundaries around a 'self' experienced as fragile or absent, and of anorexia as a two-stage process, both of which we saw in Lawrence's work, are central, and I will return to them in depth in later chapters.

I would argue, however, that there are fundamental confusions in Orbach's analysis, which stem from her attempt to present a simultaneously psychoanalytic and sociological explanation. As we have seen, Orbach notes what she terms 'the tension that exists between the two modes of inquiry – the outside and the inside, the sociological and the psychoanalytic' (ibid.: 76). But if we look further we see, I would suggest, not so much a 'tension' as an irreconcilability. As Roger Gottlieb points out: 'psychoanalytic theory takes as its goal the explanation of adult behaviour by reference to unconscious processes formed in early childhood' (quoted in ibid.: 105). A sociological understanding of psychology, on the other hand, has as its task the theorization of 'the manner by which the outer is reproduced in the inner, the way social structures become mental ones' (ibid.: 107).

Orbach tries to maintain the view that the 'integrated ego' is the gender-neutral goal of psychological development *in tandem with* the feminist argument that 'psychologies are gender-specific', and this confuses both her analysis and her therapeutic conclusions (1986: 108; 29). To provide a thoroughgoing feminist analysis of anorexia needs more than simply 'adding on' the feminist perspective to existing psychiatric orthodoxies. Rather, it requires that 'psychology' be seen through the framework of a feminist perspective, and I would argue that Orbach's work tends towards the former rather than the latter.

To pursue these arguments, I shall look at the three main areas which I see as illustrative of the basic confusions in Orbach's analysis: the constraints which the therapeutic aim places on analysis; the issue of the social construction of biological 'needs'; and the tension between the concepts of the social construction of psychology and the 'universal' self.

While I am not, as I argued earlier, taking up an 'anti-therapy' position, I would suggest that analysis with a therapeutic aim can too easily disregard the symptom itself and its meaning in the search for 'underlying causes'. This is perhaps the main difference between this thesis and Orbach's, as the exploration of the anorexic process in Part III will, I hope, show.

A therapeutic aim pushes the theorist in the direction of presenting anorexia as 'curable' on the individual level. Orbach does argue that political struggle as well as individual therapy is needed if the social structure which produces anorexia is to be changed. However, collective feminist action is heavily downgraded in favour of encouraging individual anorexic women to 'accept their needs' (ibid.: 141–57, 179–80, 192; see also Haw and Parker, 1977). Again, I'm not saying that this is not worthwhile and necessary, but it is a great deal more problematic than it appears to be here, and it is only on her last page that Orbach seems to recognize this (ibid.: 192). For example, how is the ex-anorexic woman who accepts and acts on her desires as legitimate to deal with a patriarchal society which emphatically does not? In her 'Afterword' Orbach seems to suggest that such acceptance will proceed 'naturally' from what she calls the extension of the scope of women's lives (ibid.: 192), but she gives no clues as to how this is to be achieved. This neatly sidesteps the reality of patriarchal power, the profound depth of change any feminist transformation of society would necessitate, and the likelihood of resistance to such change.

Further, although she argues that anorexia should be seen not as pathology but as on a continuum of attitudes to food and the body shared by all women, she goes on to undermine this position by re-presenting, albeit in more understanding format, the idea of the pathology-causing mother, so famed in psychiatric ideology (ibid.: 24, 48). In her suggestion that the therapist-as-good-mother can 'undo' the underlying causes of anorexia by a positive presentation of female desire, we are again working on the assumption that mothers 'cause' anorexia, and 'correct' mothering can prevent it (ibid.: 170–9). This sits most uneasily with the argument that anorexia has social causes, *and* with Orbach's own critique of conventional psychiatric treatment of the anorexic woman as a moral child (ibid.: 186). Further, this position seems to argue that the 'legitimacy' of autonomous female desire can be subjectively accepted by women as individuals in a patriarchal culture in which such a reappraisal is a profoundly political – and dangerous – act.

As we have seen, Orbach argues that anorexic women feel a 'particularly heightened sensitivity' to socialization to femininity – they hear the culture's messages 'in quadrophonic sound' (ibid.: 19, 114). Further, the anorexic woman feels her needs more strongly (ibid.: 142). So *is* their experience qualitatively different? And if so, *how* and *why*? Is this to be laid at the door of bad mothering too? If so, how do feminists answer the contention that all that is needed is a return to good mothering? The need for a transformation of social structure becomes tenuous if some – that is, non-anorexic – women can 'balance' the tension between femininity and living independent lives (ibid.: 29). We are again teetering on the brink of individual pathology arguments which legitimate individualist solutions, teaching women how to 'balance' irreconcilable social demands rather than changing them.

The second issue I would like to look at is that of biological 'need'. In *Fat is a Feminist Issue* Orbach argues that if women were not subject to social pressure towards thinness they would attain a weight that was 'natural' to them by listening to their body tell them what and how much food to eat (1978). The suggestion here is that the body 'knows' which foods and what quantities it needs; without social interference we could regulate eating and body-shape according to these internal messages. This idea of 'natural' appetite existing outside of the social is also assumed in *Hunger Strike*. For example, Orbach argues, as we have seen, that because of the objectification of the female body in modern Western culture women cannot have 'an unmediated or purely physical relation to their bodies' (1986: 36). She argues too that the body has 'basic physical needs that arise quasi-independently', needs which, if their 'internal cues' were 'correctly interpreted' in childhood would be unproblematic in adulthood (ibid.: 91, 81).

What she assumes here is that *without* such objectification, or 'wrong' interpretations, unmediated physicality is possible. We must assume that for men, and perhaps for properly brought-up women, this is how they experience their bodies. In Chapter 5 I shall develop the notion of the body as a social construction rather than a simple biological given, but briefly here I would argue that if we look at the body sociologically, seeing that both social conceptualizations and subjective experiences of the body change historically and differ for different social groups, the idea of a purely physical apprehension of the body, and of purely physical appetites which exist outside history and social structure, becomes tenuous (see Swartz, 1985; Diamond, 1985). I will argue that it is not that men have a 'natural' relationship with their bodies and their physical 'needs' and that sexism prevents women having the same, but that men's needs and women's needs, men's bodies and women's bodies, have different meanings in a patriarchal culture.

The concept of the body as a self-contained psychosomatic unity which expresses itself through manipulation of the outer environment around its own desires is, I would argue, the dominant body-concept of our culture and, as one would expect in a patriarchal culture, is phallocentric. For women such psychosomatic harmony does not exist, for the dominant body-concept coexists, for women, with the 'sub-text' of femininity. In this, women's selves, as well as their bodies, are objects in the masculine environment, and their 'boundaries' are fluid and penetrable rather than self-contained and invasive. This, I would argue, is the source both of women's 'problems' with the body and men's ease in it. Arguing thus, we can reject the notion of a supposedly more 'natural' masculine apprehension of physicality as well as the presentation of this natural physicality as the proper goal of 'maturity'.

I would argue, then, that no experience of the physical is possible 'outside' of social categorizations, definitions and imagery. For now, I would point to the acceptance of natural, gender-neutral and ahistorical biological needs by Orbach as illustrative of the lack of sufficiency and depth in her feminist critique of psychiatric ideas. It is not only psychologies which are gender-specific; the experience of physical needs is too.

Finally I would like to focus on an unexplicated confusion between the notion of the self as a social construction and the idea of a 'natural' self – of 'human nature' – in Orbach's work on anorexia. We have seen that Orbach argues that psychology is socially created; and in her discussion of the mother–daughter relationship she begins with the caveat that this model of parenting and her comments on it are 'time and culturally specific' (1986: 42, 58).

I would argue, however, that this historical and sociological focus simply does not go far enough – it is added on to rather than integrated with the psychoanalytic slant of her work. It seems that it is only *female* psychology which is truly a social creation – the masculine self remains the invisible and unanalysed standard against which the 'problems' of the insecure female self are measured, and, I would argue, the goal of therapy. Orbach argues that the 'individual psyche absorbs and interprets cultural values' and implies, therefore, that the psyche, at least in 'embryonic' form as 'the truncated person' exists *outside of* culture, which affects the self but does not construct it (ibid.: 128, 130). She sees the concept of a self organized around a core of needs and desires which it satisfies through exploitation of 'the facilitating environment' as both gender-neutral and ahistorical and, thus, a desirable goal. This is what the anorexic woman – and all women – would be if their 'psychosomatic devlopment' were not 'stunted' (ibid.: 148).

A more sociological perspective, however, would suggest that this conception of the self, and the related conception of the body, is far from the 'natural' result of 'correct' psychological development. If we argue that the self-contained self is explicable only in the context of bourgeois individualism in which the 'individual' is masculine and the environment is there to be used and manipulated, we can see that women cannot simply *decide* to attain this form of subjectivity, since one of the conditions of its existence is the construction of a receptive female psychology and body-concept as its 'opposite'. Women are *part* of the 'facilitating environment' as objects through which the masculine subject expresses itself. Women do not, as Orbach argues, 'deny' selfhood; rather, it is denied them by patriarchal social relations. The anorexic ritual, in attempting to create the body as an impenetrable barrier through control of intake, is a response and a resistance to those relations.

Women's receptive psychology is not, then, a result of 'incorrect' development but is a result of the social control of women in patriarchal culture. And in focusing so heavily on the mother–daughter relationship, Orbach 'psychologizes' and domesticates the social control of women, using much the same arguments as Chernin, albeit in more sophisticated form. Personality is not created in one relationship, but through *all* social relations. There is little point in replacing the isolated Oedipal triangle floating in unsocialized ether with an equally isolated mother–daughter dyad (see Deleuze and Guattari, 1977; Gottlieb, 1984). It is not just mothers who do not meet daughters' needs appropriately; rather, those 'needs' are socially unacceptable and threaten patriarchal order.

I would argue that anorexia, and feminine psychology in general, is better analysed *fully* sociologically. The idea of a mechanical transmission of culture by the mother is partial, an abstraction which can too easily be seen as reality. Other relationships with women and, crucially, the effect of relations with men in general, and the institution of heterosexuality in particular can all too easily disappear. Orbach concentrates on mothers' socialization of daughters into a denial of desire but does not consider sufficiently why such denial is necessary and how it is maintained outside of the mother–daughter relationship.

As Gottlieb points out, infantile experience – in Orbach's case, the experience of the mother–daughter relationship – 'takes its social meaning from its place in an overall system of social relations' (1984: 111). He argues: 'the experience of a child up to age two or three would be a great deal less important were it not reinforced throughout the rest of his or her life' (ibid.: 116). Mothering, then, is 'at most . . . *part* of the process by which male domination reproduces itself', rather than 'the primary cause of patriarchy' (ibid.: 117, 94).

Orbach, I would argue, accepts too readily the psychiatric frame of reference, and fails to take the feminist critique of gender-roles far enough. Both these features of Orbach's thesis undermine what is otherwise a fine piece of work.

CONCLUSION

The work of Orbach, Lawrence and to a lesser extent Chernin represents a major theoretical advance on the psychiatric definition of anorexia as individual pathology. All three writers locate anorexia within culture, and point to continuities in their relationships to food and the body between anorexic and non-anorexic women. Further, the concepts of desire and dependence which appeared so obliquely in the work of Crisp *et al.* are given a much more thorough discussion and are placed definitively centre-stage by Orbach and Lawrence.

I have argued, however, that this theoretical advance is partial, and that it is hampered by an incomplete acceptance of the social construction of the self and the body and consequently of the place of the gender division in physicality and subjectivity. Without a sociological analysis of the construction of desire and the body as gendered within a specific cultural context the anorexic symptom, I would suggest, can make only partial sense. Such an analysis will be pursued in Part III.

The theoretical issues involved in a sociological analysis of anorexia are, however, complex, and are more easily grasped if we have some idea of how anorexic women themselves perceive their bodies, their appetites and their illness. The following chapter, then, outlines the central anorexic meanings.

Part II

Anorexic meanings

Chapter 4

Anorexic meanings

LUCY

Lucy is now 18. She was anorexic for one year between the ages of 15 and 16, and now considers herself recovered. Her background is middle class.

I suppose it started around January/February 1985, and it got gradually worse through the whole year . . . It happened when I was 15, 16, you know, and it was a real crucial time as far as school was concerned, right in the middle of my O-levels. I mean I sat through my O-levels weighing about 5 stone, and I managed to get 7 As and a B, you know, I just can't understand how . . . I gave my school a shock, because I was sitting my O-levels looking like nothing on earth basically . . . I just wanted to be thinner and it just got out of hand.

I went on a diet, you see, and well it just went too far . . . It's a very fine balance and if you go too far you really aren't responsible for what you're doing, you lose control . . . I started to eat sort of less, sort of cut down to a certain level, and as I managed – because, you see, as you eat less and less your stomach actually shrinks and so eventually, if you're persistent enough, what you do eat makes you feel full, so you think, 'Oh, I ought to eat less', and you just go on like that . . . because your stomach does shrink. I mean when I went in [to hospital] my stomach was about the size of a walnut.

Initially when I went on the diet, I mean it was a *success*, it *worked* and I thought, hey, this is brilliant . . . I would have a piece of toast for breakfast, and to begin with I had sort of a sandwich and fruit for lunch, but then eventually I cut out the sandwich, and then when I got home from school, I would have something like a boiled egg and a piece of bread, something like that, baked beans on toast, something that would be classified as pretty light, but that would be it really, apart from perhaps – I used to have hot milk before I went to bed, but that would be it really . . . that was in the week days, during the week I was in school, so that was moulded round the school day, but at the weekends I tended to eat a bit more, I used to eat with the family, sort of Sunday roasts and things like that, and that was at the beginning. I just started to eat *less* of everything.

Sweets were the first to go, and chocolate I suppose. After that for a long while it was just sort of small amounts of everything . . . I was eating tiny bits, right up until about the day before I went into hospital, but the weight was just falling off . . . I mean at home, we eat very – healthily, is that the word? I just sort of had little bits of everything – I remember once mum cutting up sausage into tiny little bits so that I could eat it, I was just like a little baby . . . I'd try and get a bit of porridge down me for breakfast, with some milk and some brown sugar on, something like that. I don't know how much, it's very blurred . . . Sort of bits of bread with Marmite on – I had glucose, you know that powdered glucose you can get? Sort of stir that into a drink, lemon squash or something . . . If I could avoid it I would, but if my mother approached me with the drink, I wouldn't say – well, in the last day I probably would have said no, but generally I took it because I knew it was right, I mean I'm not thick, I was just ill . . . To begin with I ate on my own, so that no-one would see how little I was eating, but eventually my parents wised to it and realized that I wasn't eating much at all, and I ate with them . . . you lie, you don't mean to but you just *do*.

Once I'd eaten I'd feel really full, because my stomach was so small, but I wouldn't start to get hysterical about it, really. I would sometimes get a bit upset, because I felt so full – because nobody likes feeling bloated and full, and my parents couldn't understand how I could feel bloated and full on half a sausage and a mouthful of potato and three peas, but I really did. I mean I don't know whether I *was* full, but my mind was telling me I was over, and my mind was so locked in that it convinced me.

I wanted to be a dancer, and I wanted to lose weight . . . it was because of the dancing, I was prancing around in a leotard which shows everything anyway . . . so I did, I lost about half a stone and it looked really nice, I looked really good, it was great, I mean I lost it off my thighs and my bottom and it was just right and I should have stopped just there, because I wasn't anywhere near anorexic at that point, I looked fine, but – I don't know what made me go on, something, I just don't know.

I never used laxatives, I never used diuretics either, I just stopped eating . . . early on in the diet, I would feel really good . . . I would have a preconceived idea of what I would have in the day, and some days I would be so hungry, I was hungry to begin with, not eating so much, [and] some days I did have an extra piece of bread or something like that and think it was the end of the world . . . I was *starving*, I really was hungry, but I just had so much will, I'm a very wilful person and I just had so much willpower I just fought it all the time until it went, and it did, it did eventually.

It was a struggle, it was like a sort of internal struggle, I knew that I should have been eating, but again there was this other force, mind, whatever you want to call it that was telling me, 'No, I don't need it', and eventually the thing telling me not to eat it, the thing inside me saying not to eat, took over completely, sort of blocked out any sense of reasoning at all . . . I did try to [start eating], but half-heartedly, I was too entrenched in it really, too engulfed by the whole sort of – it just overtook me. I mean once I'd – I did make a few attempts at trying to [and] I found I just couldn't, and that was the beginning of the realization that I needed some help, to suddenly find that I couldn't do what I wanted, because this was the essence of it for me really, that I was doing what I wanted and I felt in control . . . but when I wanted to eat more again, I *couldn't*, and that upset me, because I want to be able to do what I want, I like to feel that I can, but I couldn't, and it was quite upsetting.

Throughout the whole [time], especially in the last few weeks I was at home before I went into hospital I was continually being told, look at what you're doing to yourself, you're killing yourself, and I ignored it, really, because I was so ill . . . It surprises me how long it took to connect that *I* had it. I remember someone saying to me once, before I got really bad, 'Gosh, you've lost a lot of weight, better watch it, you'll go anorexic', and I remember saying, 'Oh, what a joke' . . . It took me a long time to realize that I had it, because part of the illness is to try and ignore the fact that you are ill and carry on, no matter how thin or light you become. I didn't actually start admitting that I needed some help until I was pretty ill, you know. It took a long time . . . But then towards the end I began to feel – you can sort of block it off, it's like if you have a bad cold, you can carry on, and ignore it, and just carry on and go out and do whatever you're doing – that's what I was doing with the anorexia, but eventually I just became so ill that I couldn't ignore it in the end. I remember lying in bed, I think it was the night before I went into hospital and I just felt so *ill* . . . it hurt to lie in bed because my bones were sticking out – just the most awful feeling . . . At that point I realized I needed help, and I didn't really want to die. Because I was, I was dying.

I couldn't eat, I just couldn't eat. I got to a point where I wanted to, actually, because I knew I was ill, and I wanted to – I just *couldn't*, I can't explain it, I just *couldn't* . . . I felt very out of control, because the weight was just dropping off me . . . Alright, you did start it, but once you get past a certain point, it is uncontrollable, and you aren't responsible for your own actions.

I went down to about 4½ [stone] which was just not on, you can't cope with it at home, when you're that weight, so I had to go to hospital . . . I just lost so much weight that I had to go into hospital to have it put back on . . . about early July [1985] I went into hospital for four months . . . it was my decision. I went to the hospital, the physician examined me, and my parents came too. He spoke to me all the time, he didn't really talk to my parents, but my parents were there at that point. He said 'You're very ill and you need to come into hospital and you can either come in here', and he described what he was going to do if I came in, put me on a nasal-gastric tube, blah blah blah, or I could go back home, and if I went back home I would have been put in a psychiatric hospital. I didn't really think of it, you know, 'I don't want to go to a psychiatric hospital' – I was just so *weak* at that time, I just didn't want to go anywhere else, I just wanted to stay in that hospital, I didn't want to go any where, so I just said, 'I'll stay here'.

He explained *exactly* what was going to happen if I came in . . . he said, 'We'll tell you everything that happens, what we're doing, but you must do as we say, as far as the drip is concerned. But as far as eating is concerned', he said, 'you can eat as much or as little as you want.' If I didn't eat anything then they'd just put me on a full-strength drip all the time, and if I did eat, and put on weight they would gradually reduce the drip because I would be able to manage by myself.

When I was first admitted, I couldn't eat at all, so I had a nasal-gastric tube and I was drip fed with highly concentrated stuff, but it was diluted to begin with, a quarter strength, then gradually it was half strength and then full strength. And then as I got stronger the amount was increased, and then as I put on weight the amount was decreased, because as I put on weight I began to feel I could manage to eat again. So first of all I had the drip, because I was totally dependent on it, but then as I managed to eat more I could have my drip fluid reduced. But I had my drip throughout the whole time I was in hospital really, apart from the last week.

At first I was pretty relieved actually [to have the drip]. But I did get frustrated because – I was still ill, I was still ill in my mind when I came out of hospital, I still, you know, thought I was fat . . .

Because I've got to understand that I was *very* weak and I wasn't aware, and as I put on weight it was like waking up, it was like coming out of a deep sleep, well not a deep sleep – everything was a bit blurred, [and] still remains a bit difficult to remember . . .

When I was in hospital I used to feel – all the old ladies or other people in the ward would say, 'What's wrong with her?' You know, because I was so thin, cheekbones were out to here, bones were out everywhere really, and the drip was down me . . . They'd find out some way or other – well, perhaps they wouldn't find out, but I felt threatened – hunching over what I was trying to eat, and getting as far back in my chair near the wall as possible so no-one would see . . .

There was this one old lady on the other side of the ward and she was talking to one of the others in a loud voice, going on about this girl on the other side of the ward, going through my whole sort of eating, what I'd eaten that day and I just felt – that destroyed me for a couple of days, when my parents next came in to see me I was in tears . . .

Another thing I had to do in hospital was write down how much I ate. So when the consultant came round – he used to come round three times a week – he used to look and see . . .

When I started to eat in hospital, I started on porridge, and soup, and that was it. It was pushed forward by the nurses to a certain extent, pushing forward things that were – easy to get down, you know . . . I mean you don't have to chew them, do you? . . . [They] weren't too sort of frightening, because food frightened me. Every time – you know these big metal food trolleys – every time they came into the ward in the first two weeks I used to just burst into tears, it just caused me so much stress and upset. So it was soup and porridge to begin with, then sandwiches with the crust cut off, that sort of thing. I mean, you really go back to being a little baby. That's the way I tackled it.

Of course I got frustrated. I remember bursting into tears once just after I'd had my tea on the ward, 'I've eaten too much, I've eaten too much', and the nurse would say, 'Of course you haven't', and would calmly get this chart out and show me that I was *well* below average weight and that I really ought to eat a bit more anyway. [That was] reason coming back into it . . .

When I reached about 6 stone I was sent to a psychiatrist . . . once a week I would . . . have a chat with him. At first I hated him . . . he was trying to get me to realize why I'd done it, and I didn't like that at all. And I felt he was sort of probing into my personal life, you know, he was asking me about my family and everything and I didn't like it at all. But there again, you see, I was ill, I was hypersensitive to those sort of questions. But eventually, you know – we parted the best of friends.

One of the great boosts for me actually in my recovery was to get my O-level results, because I suddenly realized, 'Hey, I've done something good.' Because I remember the doctor came round the day the results came out and said to me 'Of course you realize that you've probably failed them all' . . . when I told the doctors they were really amazed. It was just brilliant, and it gave me quite a bit of a buck up, it was really good.

The first really good thing about it was that I wasn't in a psychiatric ward . . . I went into this general medical ward which was much better – I mean I've no experience of a psychiatric ward, but just from reading about other people's experiences, it sounds horrific.

At the beginning the nurses wrote down what I was eating, and then I took over myself because they began to trust me, I suppose. Again, I was pretty unusual in there because I didn't become very devious, or – I mean I know a lot of anorexics do, and are throwing food away, but I tried to be honest, and eventually I was doing my own drip as well, getting the cartons out of the fridge and filling it up . . .

It was acute, but it wasn't chronic, I was a lot more receptive to the treatment and didn't want to fight it, I was just very lucky.

I did improve a bit in hospital, I mean I had to, otherwise if I hadn't I would have left hospital and just stopped eating again. When I left hospital I was sufficiently well enough to realize that I had to eat . . . I considered it [not eating], but I knew that it was just, it wasn't on.

My reaction to coming out of hospital was 'Gosh, I'm so glad to come out of hospital. I'm going to really try and eat enough to keep myself out of hospital and to persevere.' When I came out of hospital it wasn't uphill all the way, I've got to admit, I did lose quite a bit of weight but not so much as to put me back in. I nearly did but not quite . . . It was quite a threat to me for a while.

I was ill in my mind, yes, when I came out of hospital it was a constant battle with reason and my sick mind, because my sick mind was saying 'You don't need to eat, you don't need food', and my – reason would come back and would say to me, 'Of course you must, because you can't survive without food.'

It was quite strange actually because my mind seemed to heal or get better as I was losing weight after I was out. I still can't understand it now. It was very strange – I think it was just down to stress and the different environment, coming from hospital . . . when I came out and was walking around a bit more active and going to school I lost a bit of weight, I ate about the same but I still lost it, because if you increase your activity level then you're going to, but the problem was that I didn't have any appetite, so I had no incentive to eat any more to compensate, but eventually my goodness it came.

When Lucy came out of hospital she was very concerned with eating 'normal' portions and eating what 'normal' people ate but what was a normal portion on the plate looked enormous and she had to continually get reassurance from her parents that that *was* a normal portion. If she was helping herself to rice or potatoes, sometimes they would say, you would really take a bit more than that, but at first she just couldn't.

It took a long time, when I came out of hospital it was still an effort, and I didn't feel hungry for *months* afterwards, months and months and months.

Well, it was strange, I used to have meals, have decent meals, you know, and not feel any different from when I went to the table to when I left it. And then I would get – eventually I did get periods of hunger, real hunger, and that used to be a bit frightening in a way, because I hadn't had them for so long. I used to – I didn't panic, but I felt a bit insecure really.

It wasn't until I started to recover or try to put on weight that I started to feel revulsions against certain foods. I felt that it was wrong to eat some things.

Once I was recovering, it took me a long time to get round to meat again, a long time, and then when I actually did, it was minced meat because it was easier to get down . . . and it took me even longer to get round to puddings and things.

It happened so slowly. I mean you don't wake up one day and think, 'I like food', it happens so slowly that you don't realize it's happening until suddenly you realize – suddenly you just think, 'Oh good, it's suppertime', and suddenly you think, 'Gosh, I just said good, it's suppertime.' It's like training yourself again . . . becoming anorexic is losing one of the basic functions, animal functions, animal instincts of being hungry, and this is why I think it's something physical that must trigger it, because it's a basic innate response, isn't it, inborn, and you actually train yourself out of it, and training yourself back into it is very hard. This is why some people die, because they just haven't the willpower to train themselves back – OK, you need willpower to become anorexic, but you need about 100 times more to come out of it again . . . Only *you* can do it, you see. They can't do it for you. You have to want to do it as well.

I didn't want to go back into hospital and I didn't want to become so ill again, because I had my school-work to get on with, and I began to realize that life wasn't that bad after all, and it was worth living.

I still want to put on some weight . . . I haven't had any periods yet . . . I'm a bit worried about the fact that I haven't had a period since February 1985 . . . They'll just come back eventually because I will put on weight, I know it will happen, but again you see it's really slow, and you just have to be patient with yourself. The slower it happens, the more likely the weight will stay on. If I go out with the specific aim of putting on, I don't know, half a stone, it'll be a lot harder than just letting it happen.

I mean that's what I really want to happen, and once that happens then I'll know that I am categorically, definitely, fundamentally normal weight, you know, and that'll be it. And I know there won't be any real danger of me – well, I suppose I really ought to keep a check on it, there is the theory that once you have anorexia you'll never be the same again, and all that sort of stuff, but I don't think I'll ever slip back again, I really don't. I honestly feel that.

It wasn't a very pleasant experience, but I learned an awful lot about myself, and about other people, and about life in general, from it. [I learned] that I'm not perfect, that I do have some sort of contribution to make to the world. I mean, the whole thing of becoming anorexic is due to lack of self-esteem, I feel, because you don't like yourself very much, you want to destroy yourself, and you have to like yourself to keep yourself going. I mean you go through periods of thinking, gosh, I'm an awful person, but generally the other side wins through and you do carry on, but with anorexia you think that you're awful, and you're not worth anything to anybody . . . [it's] setting yourself such high standards that they're just impossible to attain, which is why it happens to a lot of high-achieving people who seem to have everything going for them.

I like food in general now, I mean I feel I'm totally cured – I think I've made an amazing recovery . . . [I eat] whatever I feel like really.

I mean I'm a fairly simple case to a certain extent.

Lucy describes herself as a 'simple case'; certainly her experience of anorexia neatly fits the stereotype of the anorexic woman as an over-achieving middle-class teenage dieter who 'goes too far'. Her experience also, however, encapsulates the core meanings of anorexia. In the rest of this chapter I will compare Lucy's description of her anorexic experience and her explanations of it with those of other women whose illnesses do not fit the stereotype so neatly. Here I hope to show that although every woman's experience of anorexia is shaped by her own personal biography, we can identify a set of focal experiences which define anorexia for all women.

This 'ideal type' of anorexia centres around the meanings which women ascribe to being anorexic, and central processes which all anorexic women go through. Focusing on core experiences and meanings, I would argue, better describes the anorexic experience than a stereotype which 'excludes' many women's experiences and tends to trivialize anorexia as teenage girls' excess. In this chapter, then, I will analyse the meanings through which anorexic women make (partial) sense of the illness: need and desire, power and pressure, guilt and failure. Further, the limits of anorexic explanations will be shown – most anorexic women say that although they can make suggestions, and can point to experiences which they feel are important in discussing why they became anorexic, they are, ultimately, mystified about what their anorexia actually means, or how it can be explained.

The task of Part III, then, will be to analyse how experience which is mystifying on the individual level is meaningful on the social level. I will argue that a sociological and feminist account of how women's bodies are constructed through culture – the meanings and practices which are central here – sheds new light on the anorexic experience. This chapter will show how anorexic women describe and explain their struggle with appetite; subsequent chapters will argue that the anorexic struggle has social resonances in the cultural control of feminine desire, and will take up anew the issues of desire, power and self-discipline. In the final chapters a detailed analysis of anorexic practices will be undertaken.

CHRISTINE

Christine is now 25; she became anorexic six years ago when a post-holiday diet turned, in a way she cannot understand, into anorexia. Although she has recovered, she would still describe herself as anorexic in some important ways:

> I'm cured of the worst parts of it in as much as it doesn't control my life, and I do eat, and I am a healthy weight, and have my periods back and that – but it's always at the back of your head, it's always *there*.

Christine identifies the sense of pride and and achievement as central in her anorexia:

> I didn't have a problem, because I was *happy*, because I was *thin* and I was happy . . . Everybody obviously felt sorry for me,

because everybody else knew what was wrong, but I thought I
was terrific . . . You don't feel ill, you feel terrific, you feel really
wonderful. You've got energy, the adrenaline just flows, and
the less you eat the better you feel.

On days when she ate almost nothing, she felt:

fantastic. It felt *absolutely* brilliant days like that, that's when you
had your most energy, that's when you could have run a mile,
swum a mile, done *everything*, that's when you felt best. The less
you ate the better you felt.

What made her feel so great was her ability to resist food:

Sometimes people would comment; like sometimes you'd be out
at a social event, or at a friend's, and out would come the cakes
and buns, and they'd all be sitting there eating two sandwiches
and a biscuit and I'd be there with my black coffee and they'd
go, 'Oh you're great, I wish I was like you, I wish I could say
no, but I just can't resist it'. And I'd go, 'Oh that's great, other
people have noticed how wonderful I am, that I can resist it,
and they can't.'

Her standards were very high:

I was only ever proud of myself when I'd gone for long days
and done millions of things and hardly eaten. Nothing to be
really proud about, but nothing else matters except not eating,
achieving not eating. And specially if you'd done millions of
things that day as well, because you had used up millions of
energy which means you actually knew it was coming off – what
was already there.

The satisfaction of denial was continually threatened by hunger.
Christine always felt hungry: 'you do, you deny the most *amazing*
hunger. You'd be starved out of your brain, but you wouldn't eat.'
   However, 'sometimes I got myself so hungry that I did have to
eat, I just *had* to eat'. Failing to resist brought dire consequences:

Before you were desperately trying to resist it – that was the
main thing – resist it, overcome, willpower – you had to have
willpower to fight it and control it. And when you did give in,
you felt very *bad* – it had been a struggle and you *lost* – you felt
guilty that you had given in to it, and you felt awful about
yourself, that you didn't have the strength of character or

willpower to resist – some little bit of food . . . I thought if I ever had to eat normally I would just blow up like a balloon, that I couldn't stop, that once I did start I couldn't stop, that was the main thing. So I had to not start . . . If I'd eat one biscuit, I'd eat the whole packet of biscuits . . . [I can't] eat one, say that was nice, and put it *down*.

Resisting food is a never-ending cycle; it can never be secure, the anorexic woman can't rest on her laurels because the standard of denial spirals ever downward:

You just always feel depressed because no matter how thin you get it's not thin enough, and even when I was like going down to about 6 stone, I still felt I was fat.

LINDA

Linda was diagnosed anorexic at 11, and between the ages of 11 and 13 she was hospitalized for anorexia three times. She is now 25; since her first anorexic episode she feels that she has never been in control of her eating, and she has moved between 'compulsive' eating and anorexia ever since, always being 'on the fringes of anorexia . . . whenever I start to lose weight I want to carry on losing weight – I want to capitalize on it'. At the moment, she is 'on the slide downwards again . . . the way I feel about food just now is largely controlling me'.

Linda feels intense ambivalence about her anorexia; does she control it or does it control her? Of her initial experience of anorexia, she says:

It was like my decision, or – but then again it wasn't my decision, because again, probably with all anorexics, things get out of hand, and then you can't really help your behaviour, it's just – it rolls on and rolls on and before you're really aware of what you're doing . . . it's too late, and you just can't help yourself.

During her first hospitalization she was able to exert a measure of control over her eating:

There came a point in my first hospital stay, I don't remember when, there came a point when I gave in . . . and I started to eat all the meals – fully, not enjoying them at all – and always it was an ordeal . . . I hated being in hospital, and it was my passport out . . . I used to look forward to getting out of hospital . . . because then it wouldn't be three meals a day and I had to sit down and eat them. Then I could please myself.

She came out of hospital, immediately stopped eating and soon lost so much weight that her doctor sent her back in. She was powerless to prevent this happening a second and a third time:

By that stage, as I think any anorexic would understand, you're not in control, you can't make decisions, no matter how much you want to. I didn't like being in hospital, I didn't like it at all. And no matter how much you want to stave off something that's really bad your anorexia's in control of you, you're not in control of it . . . It takes over and nothing, nothing can stop it.

At the time of the interview, Linda's ambivalent feelings about anorexia were at the forefront of her mind: on the one hand, it gives her a sense of control and power; on the other, she feels, *it* controls her, and this embarrasses and distresses her. She is unable to fit her anorexia into her concept of herself as a person:

I'm quite a strong person, I like people and I like *life*, and I am in the grips of something I don't want to be in the grips of, and I'm embarrassed about that, and when I think about it, in sort of dispassionate moments, it's such a trivial thing, it's such an unimportant thing, really, food, to have such a control over your life and your lifestyle. I mean I do understand that, I do understand that it is a total nonsense for me to be so uptight about food and what I'm eating, and to think about it so much, it's a total nonsense. But having said that, to try and stop doing it is totally impossible for me.

There are 'good' things about being anorexic:

Now my feelings are sometimes – positive feelings. Certainly I'm powerful in that I'm in control, it is a control thing, and it's me that's controlling it, my eating and my limit and all the rest, it's me in control of that and maybe in the end . . . it's about the only damn thing that you can be in control of in your life . . . I do feel good at the control that I have, I feel good when I get to the end of the day and I'm at my limit, or I'm below my limit . . . in a lot of ways this is a crutch for me, I depend on it, it's a *control*, it's a way of controlling things, it's a *power* . . . all I can say is that there's something good about being this thin.

But at the same time anorexia is profoundly *dis*empowering:

> To me it's a question of the chicken and the egg thing, in so
> many ways my food compulsion is controlling *me* . . . I've got
> such ambivalent feelings towards it, I *hate* it, but at the same
> time, I don't want to give it up because I know, if I tried to give
> it up, if I try, if I do break out and eat something, I'm totally
> miserable . . . I would be *lost* . . . just the fact that you have
> relinquished control and let this 'full feeling' happen. I feel
> again that I've relinquished the control that I had over my
> body . . . you can't control anything else, you can't control other
> people, you *can* control your own body.

VANESSA

Vanessa became anorexic at 13, but she feels that her illness only
became serious at the age of 17. Although she has always hoped
for that 'miracle cure', at the age of 29 she feels that she is in many
ways anorexic still.

The central feeling for Vanessa was guilt:

> I couldn't eat – if I ate I felt guilty. I did feel hungry, but if I ate
> I felt guilty . . . it was this guilt that made me not eat, not the
> desire to lose weight. I didn't have this driving overwhelming
> desire to lose weight. I couldn't eat because I felt guilty.

She discovered that she was anorexic when she read a 'true life
story' in the comic *Jackie* about a girl:

> who felt guilty when she ate and I said to my mum that's the
> way I feel. Because I couldn't put into words the terrible way I
> felt when I ate anything.

At first she could cope with these feelings, but this changed when
she was 17; she remembers one particular occasion:

> I watched what I ate all the time. I hardly ate sweets or anything.
> I never ate cakes. And this night I didn't feel hungry and I didn't
> think I'd have any tea. But I ate an orange, and I felt really
> guilty after I'd eaten this orange. So I went and made myself
> sick. But I'd been making myself sick since I was 14, now and
> again. Once in a while I'd think, that was too much, I've eaten
> too much and I felt that bad about it, this terrible, terrible guilt
> if I felt I'd eaten too much I'd go and make myself sick . . . I just

would feel the compulsion to make myself sick and I'd feel better afterwards. But this night it was a driving, overwhelming guilt to make myself sick, I *had* to make myself sick.'

She was distressed by the effect her anorexia had on her family, and tried to eat, but quite simply could not: 'It was awful hard to sit and see them all crying, and begging me to eat.' When hospitalization was first suggested her family thought that this threat would be enough to make her eat:

I went to bed and my Aunt Mary came up and said, 'Will you not eat now?' And I said 'Aunt Mary I can't.' They thought that that would be enough and I would promise, but I just couldn't.

Medical intervention changed her behaviour to a certain extent. After her first hospitalization she was treated as an out-patient on a weekly basis; the appointments were on Wednesdays:

I used to go on the Wednesday, so from the Wednesday to the Saturday I hardly ate a thing, and then on the Sunday I would kind of buck my ideas up a bit and try and eat a bit for the Wednesday. I'd come out of there on the Wednesday and feel as though I'd done my bit for the week, and I deserved to have like a rest – a reprieve.

Eating was always an activity fraught with anxiety and guilt; starvation was much preferable:

It was much easier for me not eating . . . I felt more in control when I didn't eat, as if I was managing my life better . . . I felt in control, I could do what other people couldn't . . . I liked feeling empty . . . I hated having food inside me, I always associated not having food with feeling clean and pure.

What was absolutely crucial was resonsibility; did she choose to eat or did she have to? In the hospital although eating was an ordeal:

The guilt wasn't so bad because I felt they were making me eat. So I felt OK about that, because someone was always watching me when I ate . . . I couldn't eat unless I was told to eat . . . I was *glad* they didn't leave me alone, because there were a couple of times they did leave me alone and I didn't hide the food and I felt *so* guilty. I remember getting hysterical on Saturday afternoon because the nurse left me alone with soup and I ate the soup.

The real distinction was between food eaten for pleasure and food eaten because it is *needed:*

> I remember I had this desire for somebody to show me how the body worked, and to show me that the body did need food, because I didn't seem to be convinced it did need food. I used to think that it could go without food, and I wanted somebody to show me the systems of the body and how it really needed food.

ANNA

Anna is 38; she became bulimic at 30, and for the past three years has swung between anorexia and bulimia. Her eating, she feels: 'consumes your whole life, it's not just a part of your life, it is your whole life'.

Anna identifies two kinds of pressure on her. First, she feels that other people's behaviour impinges on her behaviour. She worries about her family worrying about her, 'plus I was under pressure from them to *eat* . . . the conversation would revolve around trying to get me to eat, and I found that a great pressure'. In a recent relationship with a man whom she had told about her eating he was 'very very protective and to me was becoming like my personal jailor, and protecting me from myself . . . I felt trapped, I felt caged up and that . . . control was being taken away from me.'

But the main pressure on her self-control comes from within, from appetite. Anna distinguishes between hunger and the pre-binge urge – you don't have to be hungry to binge: it is 'a 'compulsion', an 'addiction', a 'lust for food': 'nothing will stop you, nothing, you're like [a] wild animal'. The point is not simply to control the binge, but to control the 'temptation to do it':

> you think, 'I must stop this now, because if I do it again I'm not going to control it ever again, it'll take control of me and hold on to me for . . . life.'

Afterwards the shame is dreadful: 'self-*disgust* and recriminations'. Being caught in a binge:

> is as though you had been caught in murder . . . [you feel] *so guilty* so terribly guilty, I'd nearly faint with guilt at having been caught . . . the depression afterwards is absolutely – it really is

nightmarish, and I think if you have suicidal tendencies, that's when you'll do it.

She can't eat the food she really likes – 'forbidden food' – because if she ate one biscuit, one square of chocolate, she'd eat them all: 'it's like one drink to an alcoholic'. Alcohol itself is out – 'it would weaken my resolve' – that is, the resolve not to eat. When her resolve holds, she feels in control; the less she eats the more in control she feels. Trying to control her bulimia – increasing her control by eating progressively less – is Anna's explanation of how she became anorexic: 'inside every bulimic is an anorexic fighting to get out'.

She eats as little as she possibly can and then she feels proud, in control and 'more at peace'. She feels that anorexia means controlling food, and bulimia means food controlling you. If she eats a strictly planned and controlled amount of food because she knows she needs some nourishment to live, that is acceptable; if she eats because she's hungry that means loss of control:

> I think that the central word is control. When you are in control, everything else around is – the quality of your life feels much better when you're in control of whatever eating disorder you have. Whether it's anorexia, you're starving yourself, you're in control over it, you're happy. When it's bulimia, you're not bingeing, you're in control over it, you're happier . . . when you're not in control . . . you hide away, you become a recluse, and your whole life is centred on this, trying to gain control, and in doing so, trying to control that, I feel I cannot control other parts of my life, and I feel awful. When I am in control I am walking a tightrope without a net – when I binge, I fall off and there's no safety net there. And I feel everything else just disintegrates round about me, my whole life disintegrates round about me, my work, my personal relations, everything falls to pieces.

DEIRDRE

Deirdre would describe herself as a bulimic; she is now 25 and was 13 when her bulimia started, although she would not, at that age, have called it bulimia: 'I just knew that there was something wrong with the way I looked at food.' She doesn't understand 'at all' why she became bulimic, and feels totally at a loss to control or end it.

She identifies three distinct stages in her eating behaviour: the binge, starving herself after the binge to 'make up' for what she's eaten during it, and eating 'normally' in between the binge and starve cycle. The main feelings which characterize the three stages are guilt and shame when she's bingeing, control and recompense when she's starving, and a partial control coupled with dread of the next binge in between:

> You go through stages of being fine for a couple of weeks, and then I go and have a real bad binge, and that puts me down and I think well what's the point in even trying, I'm just going to slip back.

Christmas and Easter are particularly difficult times:

> Well I fall down like at Easter, people buy me Easter eggs, and at Christmas, and birthdays, and meals out for different celebrations, I fall down then. I mean Christmas is absolutely hopeless, you get boxes of chocolates, and if I've got four boxes of chocolates I would eat them all in the one go, I just couldn't keep them. And if I've a packet of biscuits, I've got to eat the whole packet, I can't just eat, you know, two.

During a binge, she does 'disgusting things' and thinks, 'oh, you horrible person'. She eats in secret, and although she would consider telling close friends about her illness, the idea of anyone seeing her bingeing, or seeing 'the results . . . two chocolate cakes and three tins of beans missing that were there . . . an hour ago', is insupportable.

The central feelings of the binge are *self-hatred* and *disgust*:

> I hate my body, I hate *myself* for being so weak and going out and buying five bags of chips and eating them, I can't be stronger and resist . . . I don't need these five bags of chips, I'm well fed, I'm healthy, I've got extra weight I could lose, I mean – I just *hate*, hate my body for a start, and hate myself for giving in to it, and wish I was stronger and could control it.

But she can't control it: 'I just sort of – have an *urge* . . . oh, I've got to have this . . . it's not *hunger*, it's just an *urge*.' The urge to get food is stronger than her willpower, her eating is in control of her. She's decided 'so many times' to stop and 'then just slipped back'.

So Deirdre recognizes that she cannot control her bulimia, and sees it as in control of her; in spite of this, she blames herself for 'slipping back', and after a binge she eats nothing at all for a certain length of time:

> I would work out how much I'd had, and I'd say well maybe that's, maybe a day and a half's worth of food, so I'll starve for a day and a half, and cancel it out that way.

When starving she feels good, that she is at least partially in control:

> And the longer I can starve the more chuffed with myself I can feel, 'cos then I feel in control, whereas when I'm bingeing I feel, oh, you've got no control, you're a useless person. When I'm starving I feel great, I feel that I'm on top of myself.

She envies anorexic women: 'it's to do with the *control*, they've got more control, they can starve for a long time and get as thin as they want'.

So for Deirdre eating is a secret cycle of discipline and strength – getting 'on top of' her appetite – and chaos and weakness – 'slipping back'; a cycle which she feels is out of her control but still her responsibility. The 'urge' to eat is overwhelming, unstoppable, and 'disgusting' in its effects. It is part of her and yet not part of her. Except for the tenuous periods of 'normality', eating veers between all and nothing; between the virtue of starvation and the shame of appetite.

Part III

The anorexic body

Chapter 5

The sociology of the body

In earlier chapters I argued that anorexia is best understood as an attempt to articulate, at the level of the body, contradictory cultural expectations of women, and that we must therefore analyse anorexia in the context of bodily meanings. I suggested that the ways in which we perceive the self and the body, the meanings through which we understand them, are culturally constructed, and thus historical. Further, historical concepts of the self and the body contain within them the central categorizations of their culture.

In this chapter, then, the argument that our perceptions of the body are imbued with social meaning will be pursued. After outlining the fundamental ideas of the sociology of the body, I will go on to analyse in detail historical examples of 'body-concepts', showing how social structure and body-concepts interact. Of central significance for this thesis, of course, will be the construction of the body as gendered.

The main task of the chapter will be to examine the contrasts between feudal and capitalist conceptualizations of the body. I will argue that a dominant feudal body-concept, and a dominant bourgeois body-concept can be analytically isolated and shown to reflect the categories of feudal and bourgeois culture. However, resistance to cultural definitions can also be found at the level of the body, and I will also explore how 'alternative' body-concepts work with and transform dominant bodily meanings.

The first historical example, then, will be what could be termed the 'official' feudal body-concept, in which the ancient notion of the four humours is combined with medieval Christianity. This understanding of the body will be contrasted with the oppositional concept of the body which can be found in medieval popular culture.

I will then go on to look at the 'high bourgeois' concept of the body, focusing on Barker-Benfield's analysis of the male body as a 'spermatic economy' and the female body as the terrain of gynaecological exploration (Barker-Benfield, 1973; 1976).

Finally, contemporary perceptions of the body will be analysed. Here I will return to the feminist and psychiatric analyses of anorexia which formed the subject matter of Chapters 2 and 3 and excavate the concept of the body which they contain, expanding their somewhat oblique discussion of the body with a consideration of phenomenological writings on the body, sociobiological under-standings, and the ideas about the body which we can discover in the 'fitness boom' of the 1980s.

THE BODY IN CULTURE

The meaning of the body in different cultures has formed, of course, a central element in much anthropological work. In spite of this, theoretical work on the sociology of the body is, to say the least, thin on the ground. Ted Polhemus argues that Hertz and Mauss were the first to emphasize 'the relationship of the physical body and the "social body" of society' (Polhemus, 1978: 9; see also Mauss, 1973; Hertz, 1960).

Suggesting that we cannot understand the body outside of culture contradicts common-sense understandings in which our knowledge of the body is seen to arise directly and uncomplicated-ly from its physical reality. As Parveen Adams points out, in this perspective the body is 'a given entity and follows the laws [of anatomy and physiology]; our bodily experience is the perception of this pre-given entity' (Adams, 1986: 28–9). Thus, knowledge of the body varies only with the sophistication of medical technique.

As Adams argues (with Beverly Brown), in common sense: 'the body is represented as being outside any existing structure, prac-tice or discourse, [as] an *externality* registered by making the body natural or pre-social' (Brown and Adams, 1979: 36).

They point out, however, that 'nature' can only be defined in relation to the social, as 'that which is non-social', 'the other of an already existing social' (ibid.: 37, 40).

Our understandings of 'nature', then, including our under-standings of the body, depend on an opposition between nature and culture which is itself social. The sociology of the body suggests that our perception of the body is 'filtered through' the structures of knowledge which categorize social life in a particular culture. Knowledge, including knowledge of the body, is mediated through ideology, rather than being a direct description of an independently existing reality.

In 'The techniques of the body', Mauss argued that the body could be properly understood only through a 'physio-psychosociological' analysis which studies the body from the three separate perspectives of sociology, physiology and psychology. Each one of these perspectives used alone gives 'dubious explanations' which need 'the collaboration of two neighbouring sciences' (Mauss, 1973, 77, 73, 85). Following this approach, Polhemus calls for the 'integration' of physiological, psychological and sociological work on the body, so that knowledge of each 'level . . . of experience' can inform the others (Polhemus, 1978: 9). Accepting that the body must be understood socially, however, does not, for Polhemus, mean that we must 'deny the reality of its electro-mechanical-chemical physicality and its psychological individuality'; sociological understanding of the body is an addition to, rather than a substitute for, physiological and psychological understandings (ibid.: 21). He argues:

> the human body does not exist and is not understandable apart from 'the social construction of reality'. Our bodies and our perception of them constitute an important part of our socio-cultural heritage. They are not simply objects which we inherit at birth, but are socialized (enculturated) throughout life and this process of collectively sanctioned bodily modification may serve as an important instrument for our socialization (enculturation) in a more general sense. That is, in learning to have a body, we also begin to learn about our 'social body' – our society.
> (ibid.: 21)

Polhemus hopes, then, to lay the foundations for analyses of the body which operate at a more general, theoretical level, and points to the work of the anthropologist Mary Douglas as one such example (ibid.: 9–10). Mary Douglas argues that the body is a metaphor or image of society, an image whose 'main scope is to express the relation of the individual to the group' (Douglas, 1971: 389, 387). She writes:

> The body is a model which can stand for any bounded system. Its boundaries can represent any boundaries which are threat-

ened or precarious . . . We cannot possibly interpret rituals concerning excreta, breast milk, saliva and the rest unless we are prepared to see in the body a symbol of society, and to see the powers and dangers credited to social structure reproduced in small on the human body.

(Douglas, 1966: 115)

The first *sociological* 'grand theory' of the body, however, is Bryan S. Turner's *The Body and Society*, the first piece of sociology to focus directly on the body-as-concept (Turner, 1984; see also 1982). Turner argues that sociology's entirely legitimate preoccupation with the rejection of sociobiology has 'submerged' the body as an object of analysis in sociology (Turner, 1984: 31). Such a rejection should be no more than a first step; what is needed is analysis of *how* we understand the body as social phenomenon. Turner attempts to use the work of Foucault to provide the general outline of this next step. He argues that the body is both a material organism and a metaphor (ibid.: 8). He argues, following Marx, that:

nature constitutes a limit on human agency, since, as part of a natural environment, we are subject to growth and decay . . . this limiting boundary is of course both uncertain and flexible, because the limits on human 'natural' capacity constantly change.

(ibid.: 204)

The body, then, is both 'social' and 'natural'. Turner argues that Marx saw nature as independent, objective reality, but as a reality which is transformed through human labour. The concept of 'nature', like all concepts, is for Marxists historical, and as such 'can only be grasped in a specific socio-historical context' (ibid.: 241). Turner is thus arguing against the perspective which would see the body as *entirely* constructed by ideology/in discourse. He argues that this would ignore what he terms 'embodiment' – that is, the personal sensuous experience of physicality – through which personal control of the body-as-environment or 'corporeal government' is developed, and which, he argues, is 'the phenomenological basis of individuality' (ibid.: 233, 245, 251). The body is thus, for Turner, both socially mediated and individually perceived (ibid.: 251).

Although Turner suggests some level of direct individual perception of physicality, he argues that our cultural understandings of the body are dependent on social structure. Biology, then, is for Turner a socially mediated classificatory system by which bodily experience is organized, rather than an 'unmediated reality': biological 'facts' exist through classification (ibid.: 29). He writes:

> Human agents live their sensuous, sexual experience via the categories of a discourse of desire which is dominant in given societies . . . [and which] is ultimately determined by the economic requirements of the mode of production.
>
> (ibid.: 14)

Similarly, biological 'needs', seen in bourgeois society as 'natural' and grounded in the 'natural' body, are also 'thoroughly penetrated and constituted by culture', their nature, context and timing being subject to symbolic interpretation and social regulation (ibid.: 27, 39). Human biological presence

> is socially constructed and constituted by communal practices . . . biology and physiology are themselves classificatory systems which organise and systematise human experience, and they are, therefore, features of culture not nature.
>
> (ibid.: 246)

Here Turner follows and amplifies Foucault's argument that the body is an object of power, produced so as to be identified and controlled (ibid.: 35). In *The History of Sexuality*, Foucault argues: 'The classical age discovered the body as object and target of power . . . the docile body . . . [which] may be subjected, used, transformed and improved' (Foucault, 1979: 136). Turner argues that Foucault's work can be used to point to the *historicity* of the body. Power is commonly seen to repress desire, which therefore exists outside of it. For Foucault, however, power is *constructive* – desire is created by power, sexuality in modern societies being continually produced and examined in, specifically, medical and psychiatric discourses. Desire, then, is the product of specific historical discourses rather than 'a unified phenomenon' (Turner, 1984: 48). Turner argues that the same can be said of the body, but suggests that in spite of his perspective on desire, Foucault appears to see the body as 'a unified, concrete aspect of human history', a view at odds with his treatment of sexuality and desire and with the argument that the body is constructed in discourse (ibid.: 48).

Turner, then, chooses to follow what Foucault says rather than what he does. He argues against the notion that culture represses independently existing bodily needs – that there is a conflict between (rational) civilization and (irrational) physical needs and desires – and for an understanding of the body developed along the lines of Foucault's concept of desire. The body for Turner, then, is also created through discourses of power, and is created in order to be controlled (ibid.: 61–4, 83, 214). The body is a metaphor of society, and illness and disease metaphors of structural crisis. Social inequalities, Turner argues, 'are fought out at the level of a micro-politics of deviance and desire' (ibid.: 114).

The body, then, is for Turner 'both a natural phenomenon and a social product', a cultural construct as well as a biological entity (ibid.: 232). This perspective allows us to investigate and analyse the meanings contained in body-concepts, whether dominant or oppositional, in our own and other cultures, and thus provides a basic structure for sociological analyses of particular historical body-concepts.[1]

I would, however, take issue with Turner on one point – his notion of embodiment and 'corporeal government'. He argues that our sense of being in control of our individual bodies is the basis of individuality. While I would accept that the body exists objectively as well as symbolically, I would question whether the distinction between 'natural', or individually perceived, and 'cultural', or socially structured sensuous experience is quite so easily drawn as Turner supposes. His argument here seems to have something in common with Polhemus's suggestion, following Mauss, that the body has analytically discrete physiological, psychological and social 'levels'.

It seems somewhat contradictory to argue that our perception of 'personal' sensuous experience is not as much a product of culture as any other apprehension of the meaning of physicality, or to argue that physiological or psychological experience of the body can be understood outside of knowledge which is socially produced. Turner himself points out that phenomenological possesssion of the body through embodiment does not always entail ownership, especially for women, and points out that women can experience their bodies as alien (ibid.: 233–4). I would argue that here Turner undercuts his own concept of embodiment, and would suggest that 'corporeal government' depends as much on cultural as on biological presuppositions. I would question whether any 'direct' – that is, socially unmediated – physical experience is possible. This is not to suggest, of course, that the body does not physically, biologically or objectively exist: rather, *all* knowledge of, ideas about, and feelings in that 'objective reality' are constructed in ideology. This is what I understand Brown and Adams to be suggesting (1979).

It is from this perspective on the sociology of the body, and bearing in mind this difference with Polhemus and Turner, that the historical examples of body-concepts in the remainder of the chapter proceeds. It is to this that we now turn.

MEDIEVAL CONCEPTS OF THE BODY

How was the body understood in feudal culture? I want to answer this question in two parts. First I would like to look at the 'official version', where the body fits into a rigidly classified cosmology, organized around the dichotomy of soul and flesh. Then I will look at the oppositional body-concept of popular, or carnival culture, using Bakhtin's brilliant reconstruction, in which the body is celebrated as open, dynamic and regenerative.

Bakhtin argues that 'official' feudal culture 'is founded on the principle of an immovable and unchanging hierarchy in which the higher and the lower never merge', and in which 'hard, well-established lines are drawn between all phenomena' (Bakhtin, 1968: 166, 433). Within this rigid system of categorizations, it was the doctrine of the four humours which provided the immediate framework through which the body was understood. The four humours – black bile, phlegm, yellow bile and blood – were held, as Klibansky, Saxl and Panofsky explain, to correspond to

> the cosmic elements and to the divisions of time; they controlled the whole existence and behaviour of mankind, and, according to the manner in which they were combined, determined the character of the individual.
>
> (Klibansky, Saxl and Panofsky, 1964: 3, 1)

This schema, Klibansky *et al.* argue, remained in force for more than 2000 years, virtually unchanged from its ancient beginnings through the Middle Ages up to the Renaissance, with Galen as its outstanding proponent (ibid.: 10; 48; 88).

The doctrine of the humours formed the basis of physiology and later of psychology. It was based on a cosmology in which basic elements or qualities were identified, qualities through which 'the complex and apparently irrational structure of both macrocosm and microcosm could be directly traced' (ibid.: 4, 3). At every level – cosmos, body, mind and soul – four basic elements could be identified. For example, the four elements of the cosmos were earth, air, fire and water, and for the soul, intellect, understanding, opinion and perception. Equilibrium of the four qualities was essential 'to any value, moral, aesthetic or hygienic' (ibid.: 4).

In bodily terms:

> each of these four elements had to be interpreted in terms of a quality which established, as it were, an apparent link between the original elements and the corresponding components of the human body, which could not, in their empirical actuality, be regarded as pure earth, pure water, and so on . . . certain real substances which appeared to correspond to those elements and qualities had to be found in the human body, for only then could the speculations of natural philosophy be reconciled with the empirical evidence of medicine and physiology.
>
> (ibid.: 5)

We can trace the development of the doctrine of the humours from its ancient origins to the more complex form which it took when viewed through the prism of Christian theology. Empedocles had described the human body as a simple combination of earth, air, fire and water, and this categorization was modified first by Philistion, head of the Sicilian school of medicine, who argued that each element possessed a corresponding 'quality' – respectively, dryness, cold, heat and moisture. This new method led to many more differentiations, of quality as well as quantity, and allowed a categorization which was freed from direct elemental linkage while still retaining strict correspondences (ibid.: 7). In *Of the Nature of Man* (cited in Klibansky *et al.*, 1964), attributed to Hippocrates or Polybus, and written no later than 400 BC, the system was developed thus:

Humour	Season	Qualities
Blood	Spring	Warm and moist
Yellow bile	Summer	Warm and dry
Black bile	Autumn	Cold and dry
Phlegm	Winter	Cold and moist

Each humour, then, was described by two qualities with elemental relationships, and each was dominant in the body in a different season. The humours were the 'surplus' left over after food had been converted through the digestion – what was indigestible. Blood, of course, did not fit this description of a surplus humour. The theory of the humours, in fact, depended on 'two quite arbitrary assumptions' – the inclusion of blood in the system, and distinguishing bile, previously seen either as one single fluid or split into numerous categories, into two types: yellow and black (ibid.: 9, 8). Each humour was situated in a different place in the body – the brain, the heart, the navel and the phallus – and had its own means of exit – nose (blood), ears (yellow bile), mouth (phlegm) and eyes (black bile) (ibid.: 4, 58).

Further, each season was matched with one of the four ages of man – boyhood, youth, maturity and old age. Thus were connected the elements, the seasons, the ages of man, the four bodily humours, and also physical types, for, 'heat made a man tall, cold short, moisture fat and dryness thin' (ibid.: 57, 10).

Health relied on the absolutely right combination in the body of the four humours. Since each humour was held to be dominant in a specific season, and since the absolutely healthy man who was never ill at all was very hard to locate, perfect humoural balance was seen as an ideal type which hardly ever occured. Most people had more of one humour than perfect harmony required, and were thus predisposed to the specific illnesses which 'their' humour caused. In Isidore's phrase, 'the healthy are governed by these four humours, and the sick suffer from them' (quoted in ibid.: 12).

The melancholy temperament, for example, related to black bile, and to air, and thus flatulence and stomach disorders were caused by black bile. The melancholy person was also said by Aristotle to be lustful:

For the sexual act is connected with the generation of air, as is shown by the fact that the virile organ quickly increases from a small size by inflation. Even before they are capable of emitting semen, boys approaching puberty already find a certain pleasure in rubbing their sexual organs from wantonness, the manifest reason being that the air escapes through the passage through which the fluid flows later on. Also the effusion and impetus of the semen in sexual intercourse is clearly due to propulsion by air . . . That they contain air is obvious in some cases; for most melancholy persons have firm flesh and their veins stand out, the reason being the abundance not of blood but of air.

(Aristotle, Problem XXX, 1, in Klibansky *et al.*, 1964: 22)

Klibansky *et al.* argue that 'what had of old been symptoms of illness came gradually to be regarded, at first unconsciously, as types of disposition'. The descriptions choleric, phlegmatic, sanguine and melancholy could mean 'either pathological states or constitutional aptitudes', and came to describe character types or psychology (ibid.: 12, 10–19).

Klibansky *et al.* refer to the work of William of Conches in arguing that it was in conjunction with Christian dogma that the idea of temperaments being determined by the humours was revived after the twelfth century: 'we might well speak of a revival of the ancient characterological doctrine within the framework of Christian moral theology' (ibid.: 106).

In William of Conches's *Philosophia* the doctrine of the humours was incorporated into Christian cosmology. He argued that when the waters receded from the earth after the Flood, moisture, fire, earth and air 'prevailed' in different places and thus the substances which created the animals arose. This resulted in, for example, choleric animals like the pig, and melancholic animals like the ox and the ass. It was only when the elements were equally proportioned that man could be created. In the Fall, however, man lost his perfect balance, 'through the privations imposed on him by life outside paradise' (ibid.: 103, 102). The animals could be melancholic, choleric or phlegmatic, but not sanguine; man, originally sanguine, due to his corruption had degenerated into the melancholic, the choleric and the phlegmatic (ibid.: 105).

This presentation of the doctrine of the humours, Klibansky *et al.* argue, served a double purpose:

first to trace the variety and inequality of men back to the Fall, which destroyed the original perfection and unity; secondly, to establish and account for the inalienable nobility of human nature.

(ibid.: 106)

The doctrine of the humours was thus fitted into Christian cosmology, and became 'part of the common stock of knowledge'. The 'popularization' of the doctrine, which took place in the fourteenth and fifteenth centuries, emphasized the link with diseases particular to each type, and how to avoid them (ibid.: 113). We can see, therefore, that the dominant or official concept of the body in medieval culture relied on a rigid system of categorizations. All of nature was explained in the one system, and the revival of the ancient doctrine of the humours through the framework of Christian ideology gave that cosmology a moral tone. Through the doctrine of the humours the body fitted into a schema in which everything had its place. As Southern argues, 'Christian medieval theology explained the purpose and place of man in the universe through its description of the cosmos', as, in Bakhtin's description, 'the narrow, vertical, extratemporal model of the world, with its absolute top and bottom, its system of ascents and descents' (Southern, 1970: 22; Bakhtin, 1968: 405). The correspondence to feudal social structure in which social positions from the king downward were fixed and immutable, and defined those who occupied them, is clear. Power, like temperament both physical and moral, was fixed, unchanging and based on God's order and the order of the cosmos. As Gurevich argues, 'social categories . . . are . . . tied up with, intertwined with, the cosmic categories in the closest possible way':

> Theology represented the highest generalization of medieval man's social behaviour; it provided a general semiological system in terms of which the members of feudal society apprehended themselves and saw their world motivated and explained . . . [It explained] the irreducible contrasts of wealth and poverty, dominion and subjugation, freedom and bondage, privilege and deprivation.
>
> (Gurevich, 1985: 14; 9; 10)

Further, medieval Christianity offered the resolution of the eventual spiritual transcendence of worldly ills; as well as explaining feudal social structure, then, it provided 'its sanction, its justification and sanctification': 'the earthly feudal system is an isomorph of the hierarchy of God's creatures and the ranks of the angels' (ibid.: 10, 70).

The body in Medieval Christianity

As we have seen, the doctrine of temperaments took on a moral character in its Christian revival – the melancholic, choleric and phlegmatic being corruptions of the original sanguine. While all phenomena in the universe were understood as having fixed places in a single structure, the structure of nature was itself defined through a fundamental division between 'the earthly world and the supernatural world' which Gurevich describes as 'the ineluctable opposition between the sublime and the base' (Gurevich, 1985: 6). Gurevich argues that the perception of all types of natural phenomena as similarly constituted – the 'belief in the unity of the universe', 'the inseparability of its various spheres', the idea of 'the microcosm' as 'a replica of the macrocosm' – coexisted with the fundamental contrasts 'of eternal and temporal, sacred and sinful, soul and body, heavenly and earthly' in the medieval Christian world-view (ibid.: 9–10, 13).

Here, Gurevich argues, we:

> have to take into account the changes which the concept of 'cosmos' underwent in its transition from the ancient world to the world of the Middle Ages. Antiquity saw the world as complete and harmonious; medieval man saw it as dualistic.
>
> (ibid.: 58)

In this opposition the body, after the Fall, was fundamentally corrupted, linked with the world rather than with heaven. Thus, the body was seen in Christian theology as the prison of the soul, the symbol, as it were, of earthly corruption.

Turner argues that in medieval Christianity the body was seen as the seat of unreason, passion and desire, and thus as the cause of sin (Turner, 1984: 36, 13). The flesh was symbolic of moral corruption which threatened the feudal order, and should be controlled by asceticism, with diet and abstinence basic elements of 'a regimen for the control of desires' (ibid.: 166, 36). The aim of ascetic regimes, then, was 'to liberate the soul from the cloying distractions of desire' (ibid.: 216).

There was no firm line drawn between sin and disease at this time, and R.J. Moore argues that an imbalance of humours not only caused illness but was simultaneously a manifestation of sin; diseases, then, 'could . . . be classified according to the sins of which they were the bodily expression' (Moore, 1976: 4). Leprosy, for example, was seen as the bodily manifestation of heresy; Moore quotes Rhabanus Maurus: 'Lepra est doctrina haereticorum falsa atque varia . . . leprosi sunt haeretici Dominum Jhesum Christum blasphemantes' (ibid.: 4). Moore points out that 'the comparison of heresy and disease provided not simply a casual or convenient metaphor, but a comprehensive and systematic model', a coherent system of understanding in which 'heresy was to the soul what leprosy was to the body' (ibid.: 9, 11).

The body and the soul, then, were intimately linked, the state of one being mirrored in the condition of the other. The best conditions for the soul were realized in monastic asceticism, in which the world and the pleasures of the flesh were renounced (Brooke, 1978: 81). Ascetic rules liberated the soul for prayer, being, in Leyser's term 'structures for piety' (Leyser, 1984: 3). These best conditions, of course, were only realizable for the few, who laboured in their ascetic withdrawal from the world as 'spiritual soldiers' on behalf of the many (Southern, 1970: 224). As Southern points out:

> the main centres of religious life in medieval Europe were communities specially endowed and set apart for the full, life-long and irrevocable practice of the Christian life at a level of excellence judged to be impossible outside such a community. The members of these bodies were known as viri religiosi: they were 'the religious' in contrast to all other men whether secular or clerical.
>
> (ibid.: 214)

Monastic withdrawal from the world was based on the idea that life in the world could not be fully holy; although since the Fall the perfect life could not be lived anywhere, the next best thing was the monastic life of discipline, prayer and self-abnegation. The world was 'either meaningless or filled with evil' and the monasteries 'replicas of heaven on earth' (ibid.: 31, 28, 341):

> they were institutions designed to stem the tide of change. The idea of a changeless society forever enshrined within the fleeting shadows of the world was written into their title-deeds and discipline . . . they were snatching a small portion from the world of meaningless change to make it a replica of eternity.

Outside there was visible aimless flux; within, the image of invisible immutability.

(ibid.: 28–9)

Within the monastery the rule was all, the individual nothing. As in the feudal order as a whole, every man had his station and was defined by it; spiritual perfection was to be sought through discipline and hierarchy (ibid.: 33, 43, 231).

Withdrawal from the world was effected through (usually) poverty, chastity and diet. Money, sex and food were therefore of the world, and Leyser tells us that although prohibitions varied, fats, meat and wine were often forbidden. Rules for fasting again varied; fasting could mean eating one meal a day, or eating only bread, salt and water (Leyser, 1984: 66). Some Orders were also more scrupulous than others in the observance of the holy poverty of Christ.

But although wealth and over-indulgence in food and drink and physical comfort as a whole were renounced in asceticism, from the feminist viewpoint the proscriptions on sex are the most interesting, for it becomes clear here that the meaning of 'the flesh' is highly gender-differentiated. While all flesh, regardless of gender, imprisons the soul, female flesh more profoundly imprisons the female soul. Further, female flesh also endangers the male soul, since women and sexual pleasure were substantially the same thing.

For St Bernard 'every woman was a threat to his chastity . . . he saw vast and nameless dangers in . . . [the] easy association of men and women' (Southern, 1970: 314). St Francis warned against 'the snares of female companionship' and in his *Life* it is claimed that he never looked a woman in the face (Brooke and Brooke, 1978: 282). Women, Smith argues, were seen as 'the instruments of temptation of the flesh', being more wicked and more lustful than men (Smith, 1978: 177; see also Southern, 1970: 311; Thompson, 1978: 227). Sheila Rowbotham writes of 'a repeated male complaint about the sexual insatiability of women' (Rowbotham, 1977: 7). And Eileen Power argues that St Paul's conception of women as the 'instrument of the Devil' was embedded in monastic ethics, philosophy and ascetic regimens. Women were 'the greatest of all obstacles in the way of salvation', 'the gate of hell' (Power, 1973: 16, 10; see also Brooke, 1978: 6; Hamilton, 1978: 52).

The sins of the flesh, then, were seen to reside principally not in male desire but in the female body, and male salvation depended on the removal of the object of temptation. *Female* salvation, unable to rely on this tactic, was a little more complicated. On the ideological level the Virgin Mary existed as an alternative ideal for women, an ideal which women could to some extent use to counter their innate evil and materiality (Power, 1973: 10). However, the monastic life depended on wealth and status, and was thus even less available for women than for men. Further, as Power argues:

> Monasticism may have offered a refuge for some women; but the refuge merely sealed the degradation of women in general by confining full approbation to those who withdrew themselves from the world.
>
> (ibid.: 16)

Those who could withdraw from the world were aristocratic women (Southern, 1970: 310), and these 'cloistered virgins', Hamilton argues, removed themselves from the world 'as objects of temptation for men' (Hamilton, 1978: 52).

These economic and ideological constraints on the religious life for women did not, however, prevent women from trying to withdraw from the world. The Cistercian Order especially attracted women, and in twelfth-century Europe there was an expansion of Cistercian nunneries established under the patronage of individual men. This expansion, Southern tells us, took place 'without the slightest notice being taken of it in the official acts of the Cistercian Order' and the nunneries had no formal position in the Order's structure (Southern, 1970: 315). Thompson points out that the Cistercians 'at first ignored and then barely tolerated the ladies who wished to share their fervour and imitate their customs' (Thompson, 1978: 242).

In fact, when the infiltration of so many women into the Order *was* offically noticed, an effort to limit and control the female incursion took place (Southern, 1970: 315–18). In the Premonstratensian Order, too, the twelfth century saw a crackdown on women. Abbot Conrad of Marchtal wrote:

> We and our whole community of canons, recognizing that the wickedness of women is greater than all the other wickedness of the world, and that there is no anger like the anger of women,

and that the poison of asps and dragons is more curable and less dangerous to men than the familiarity of women, have unanimously decreed for the safety of our souls, no less than for that of our bodies and goods, that we will on no account receive any more sisters to the increase of our perdition, but will avoid them like poisonous animals.

(quoted in ibid.: 314)

Women's vows of chasitity were not enough, then, to prevent them from being objects of temptation to their male counterparts.

Although feminine flesh was the real seat of sin, and women's inherent sinfulness was hardly eradicable even through ascetic regimens, this did not prevent women from trying – they simply had to try harder. Women could define sexual pleasure as a whole, rather than their bodies alone as the sin, and indeed Southern argues that 'disgust at the recollection or prospect of marriage seems to have played a very large part in recommending the monastic life to women' (ibid.: 311). Religious women renounced marriage, took a vow of chastity and dedicated their lives to Christ (ibid.: 326; Bolton, 1978: 256; Brooke, 1978: 5; Holdsworth, 1978: 198).

Women were allowed only a very minor role in the Church, and Southern argues that it was women's desire for a 'spiritual importance' denied them by orthodox Chritstianity which led to their strong atttraction to heretical movements. The Beguines, for example, were an all-women movement which began in Liège in 1210. Their name derives from the heretical Albigensians, and was a pejorative name given to women who rejected marriage for celibacy (Southern, 1970: 321–2). Women's quest to reject the world and the flesh on equal terms with men was attacked from both sides; neither lay society nor the Church could accept the divorce of the female soul from the female body and its desires.

We have seen in the analysis of Bell's work the lengths to which St Catherine and other female ascetics went to mortify their flesh, and that their excesses angered and perturbed their male confessors and the church authorities (Bell, 1985). B.M. Bolton also writes of Mary of Oignies' 'incredible feats of endurance in fasting, prayer and lack of sleep'. Her contemplation of the Passion 'induced in her such a loathing of her own body that she cut off pieces of her own flesh with a knife'; she was 'filled with the holy food of Christ's flesh and purified and cleansed by his life-giving blood'

(Bolton, 1978: 363, 266). And Southern quotes Mechthild of
Magdeburg:

> My body is in great distress.
> My soul is in highest bliss,
> for she has seen
> and thrown her arms around
> her Loved One all at once.
> Poor thing,
> she is distressed by him:
> he so draws and delights her,
> she cannot withhold herself,
> and he brings her into himself.
> Then the body speaks to the soul:
> 'Where have you been? I cannot bear it any more.'
> And the soul says, 'Shut up, you fool,
> I want to be with my beloved;
> You will never enjoy me any more –
> I am his joy; he is my distress –
> Your distress is, that you can no longer enjoy me:
> You must put up with this distress
> For it will never leave you.'
>
> (Southern, 1970: 327)

This feminine 'super-mortification', I would argue, can be directly
related to the concept of the female body as 'super-flesh' in
medieval Christian ideology. Although there existed sufficient
ideological ambiguity for women to try in numbers to escape the
prison of their flesh, this was an almost hopeless task, as flesh was
what defined them. Men could escape the flesh by an avoidance
of women; women were fundamentally trapped. In the extreme
physical asceticism of Catherine of Siena we can see an attempt to
purify and transcend her female flesh: since her body was, as
female, intrinsically more sinful, her efforts to escape the flesh had
to be greater than those of her male counterparts. No wonder she
so irritated her confessors with efforts which to them would have
had a continual whiff of futility about them.

The doctrine of the humours, then, seen in the context of
Christian theology, gives us a body-concept dependent on rigid
hierarchical categorizations in which the central defining dichotomy is that of body and soul, reflecting the cosmological
dichotomy of heaven and earth. As in the wider feudal culture,

only an elite few could detach themselves from the world of matter, flesh, sin and flux through ascetic regimens which brought them closer to heaven's changeless realm of spirit. Spiritual perfection and union with God was achievable only through transcending the flesh. Membership of the elite was fixed – each person had his or her inescapable place in a God-given hierarchy. And membership of the elite was gender-specific; women's bodies linked them all but irrevocably with the world.

The concept of the body in carnival culture

Although the ideological domination of the Church in the Middle Ages is often suggested – Southern, for example, argues that the church was 'a compulsory society' (1970: 17), and Roberta Hamilton argues that its views 'went almost unchallenged' (Hamilton, 1978: 50) – Bakhtin's work shows that a critique of the hierarchical power of feudalism and Catholic ideology did exist in popular culture. His study of popular carnival culture reveals both an alternative and oppositional conception of feudal social structure and a corresponding alternative and oppositional perception of the body. It is to this we now turn.

Bakhtin argues, of Rabelais, that popular sources – idioms, sayings, proverbs – 'determined the entire system of his images and his artistic outlook on the world' (Bakhtin, 1968: 2). His writing is 'non-official', in that it is isolated from literary, but at home with popular culture. This foundation in medieval popular culture, Bakhtin argues, allows us to use the work of Rabelais as an expression of that culture. He argues that in feudal societies a 'two-world condition' existed, in which the popular culture of humour and carnival scoffed at and parodied the official feudal culture. It is here that understandings of the body oppositional to that of Christian ideology can be found. The consciousness of medieval man, then, contains both carnival and Christian understandings of life (ibid.: 3, 6, 96).

As we have seen, in 'official' feudal culture, the body was analysed as occupying a fixed place in a fixed cosmos, and as the prison of the soul. In carnival culture this understanding was overturned through the essential principle of the carnival imagery of grotesque realism – degradation. Here, Bakhtin argues that the ideal and the spiritual are reduced or degraded to the material, physical level, 'the sphere of earth and body' (ibid.: 19). We must be wary, however, of seeing the degradation of grotesque realism through modern eyes. In medieval carnival imagery 'degradation' is not a negative term, but represents subsumption into 'the positive, regenerating and renewing lower stratum' in which the body:

> makes no pretence to renunciation of the earthly . . . this is not the body and its physiology in the modern sense of these words, because it is not individualized. The material bodily principle is contained not in the biological individual, not in the bourgeois ego, but in the people, a people who are continually growing and renewed. This is why all that is bodily becomes grandiose exaggerated, immeasurable . . . the leading themes of these images of bodily life are fertility, growth and a brimmming-over abundance.
>
> (ibid.: 23, 19)

Degradation or debasement did not mean simple destruction or befouling, but a *renewal* on the material bodily level in an elimination of hierarchical divisions. So for Rabelais the subsumption of the ideal/spiritual in the material was positively renewing, drawing it into the body understood as the body of the people in which death and rebirth are inextricably intertwined, into 'the fruitful earth and the womb' (ibid.: 21, 224).

There are three central points to be understood here. First, in carnival culture the hierarchies of feudal culture are overturned; the king becomes the peasant, the peasant the king, and fixed power relations are satirized. The hierarchy of body and soul was itself overturned: the body, from being the prison of the soul, becomes the locus of life and regeneration, and is celebrated rather than renounced (ibid.: 19). And second, the body in carnival culture is not individualized but represents the body of all the people, in a 'material bodily whole which . . . transgressed the limits of . . . isolation' (ibid.: 23; see also Gurevich, 1985: 53–4). It is because the body is collective that death is part of fertility and renewal rather than an absolute end and individual tragedy. Grotesque realism 'discloses the potentiality of an entirely different world' and thus 'liberates humanity from necessity' (Bakhtin, 1968: 48–9). The humour which is fundamental to it liberates the common people from fear of oppression by nature, death and of the consecrated and forbidden (ibid.: 90, 226). It represents an overturning of the hierarchies of feudal power relations in a critique of the fundamental separations which structure and justify them.

The conception of the collective body is expressed through the imagery of abundance, with 'exaggeration, hyperbolism, excessiveness' being 'fundamental attributes' of grotesque realism (ibid.: 303). The central image is the huge size and appetites of Gargantua, where images of gluttony and drunkenness express not private appetites, but the appetite for life of the people as a whole, and their triumphant absorption in their environment (ibid.: 301–2).

Third, and relatedly, carnival bodily imagery is essentially *dialectic* (ibid.: 211–12). Bakhtin argues that the carnival body is *process* rather than product:

> life . . . is the epitome of incompleteness. And such is precisely the grotesque concept of the body . . . [in which] the grotesque body is not a closed, completed unit: it is unfinished, outgrows itself, trangresses its own limits.
>
> (ibid.: 26)

The image of the body is of 'contradictory, perpetually becoming and unfinished being' (ibid.: 118, 316). Thus parts of the body open to the outside world are stressed:

> the unfinished and open body (dying, bringing forth and being born) is not separated from the world by clearly defined boundaries; it is blended with the world, with animals, with objects. It is cosmic, it represents the entire material bodily world in all its elements . . . as the swallowing up and generating principle.
>
> (ibid.: 26–7)

Since grotesque realism represents a collective body, the boundaries between body and world are seen quite differently than boundaries between the world and the *individualized* body. The grotesque focus on the body as open to the world, and as intruding into the world gives a central role to

> that which protrudes from the body, all that seeks to go out beyond that body's confines . . . all that prolongs the body and links it to other bodies or to the world outside.
>
> (ibid.: 316)

The common characteristic between bodily orifices and protrusions is that within them the divisions of body and soul, and of body and world, are overcome. Grotesque imagery ignores the closed surface of the body and concentrates on 'excrescences . . .

and orifices . . . that which leads beyond the body's limited space
or into the body's depths. Mountains and abysses, such is the relief
of the grotesque body; or . . . towers and subterranean passages'
(ibid.: 318, 317).

Grotesque language, then:

> was orientated toward the world and toward all the world's
> phenomena in their condition of unfinished metamorphosis:
> the passing from night to morning, from winter to spring, from
> the old to the new, from death to birth.
>
> (ibid.: 165)

This essentially dialectical conception of the world and the body,
Bakhtin argues, could only be expressed in 'unofficial' culture and
in opposition to and critique of the founding principle of official
feudal culture – 'an immovable and unchanging hierarchy in
which the higher and the lower never merge', in which there are
'hard, well-established lines between all phenomena', and in which
the order of the world was static, unchanging and eternal (ibid.:
106, 433). The official view could not be overcome by individual
thought, only by popular culture as a whole (ibid.: 275).

Images of bodily life – eating, drinking, copulation, birth,
defecation – were central in Rabelais's work, and express these
three central features of degradation as renewal, the body as
collective, and the body as process. As Bakhtin argues, images of
eating create:

> an extremely dense atmosphere of the body as a whole in which
> all the dividing lines between man and beast, between the
> consuming and the consumed bowels are intentionally
> erased . . . these consuming and consumed organs are fused
> with the generating womb. We thus obtain a truly grotesque
> image of one single, superindividual bodily life, of the great
> bowels that devour and are devoured, generate and are gener-
> ated. But this, of course, is not an 'animal' or 'biological' bodily
> life. We see looming beyond Gargamelle's womb the devoured
> and devouring womb of the earth and the ever-regenerated
> body of the people.
>
> (ibid.: 226)

Banquet imagery, then, represents eating not as a commonplace,
privatized and individualized activity but as a popular feast, a
'banquet for all the world' in which eating is a social event rather

than a biological act (ibid.: 278, 281). It is in eating that the body transgresses its own limits and 'is enriched and grows at the world's expense'. In eating, humanity encounters the world:

> here man tastes the world, introduces it into his body, makes it part of himself . . . [further] Man's encounter with the world in the act of eating is joyful, triumphant; he triumphs over the world, devours it without being devoured himself. The limits between man and the world are erased, to man's advantage.
>
> (ibid.: 281)

What Bakhtin and Rabelais show, then, is the 'laughing chorus' of official feudal culture, a chorus in which the body is *open, collective* and *dialectic* (ibid.: 367). The point and counterpoint of medieval concepts of the body, I would therefore argue, show how the body is understood and perceived through the framework of world-view. In the dominant understanding of the body, hierarchy and dichotomy, the central organizing principles of Christian cosmo-logy, define the body. In the oppositional carnival culture, these values were overturned, in a satire of the hierarchical social struc-tures which underpinned them. The body was seen as part of the dialectical cycle of life and death, a unitary concept of material existence which negated the dichotomies of heaven and earth, flesh and spirit.

The medieval body: flesh and super-flesh

The body-concepts of feudal and carnival culture come to us, it must be remembered, through the writings, almost exclusively, of men. We have very little material direct from women – even the *Lives* of Bell's 'holy anorexics' are women's experiences translated through masculine frameworks. It is difficult to reconstruct with any certainty how women reacted to these conceptualizations of their bodies, what acceptances, rejections or negotiations took place.

I have suggested that the devaluing of women in Christian ideology was resisted in women's insistence that they too could live the religious life and transcend the body. But the discussion of a female perspective on the medieval concepts of the body can really only be speculative. What we can identify are patriarchal under-standings of women and their bodies. I have suggested that women's bodies were defined as 'super-flesh' in theology, and I

would argue that the gender difference was expressed quantita-
tively rather than qualitatively both in Christian and in carnival
categorizations. The difference between the two concepts lies not
in the structure or form of their expression of the gender difference of bodies, but in the different value they placed on flesh
and spirit. To put it crudely, if women equal super-flesh, their
value is *decreased* in Christian cosmology but *increased* in carnival
imagery.

As we have seen, in the Christian concept the body was the
fundamental symbol of earthly corruption. The most valued spiritual path resisted physical demands and sought spiritual
transcendence – the elimination as far as possible of the earthly
and corrupt in order to approach union with the pure spirit of
God. Men and women, as we have seen, did not have equality of
access to salvation since the transcendence of the flesh was, for
women, an almost impossible task. Women, through their bodies,
were tied much more closely to the realm of earthly corruption
than were men. But this was a difference of quantity rather than
of quality: both genders were linked through their bodies to the
material realm, and for both this link was a negative one.

Conclusions about the popular view of the female body will of
necessity be more tentative. Information is scarce, and Bakhtin has
little to say on the gender division in carnival imagery. The only
sustained discussion specifically on women is his short analysis of
the '*querelle des femmes*' – a sixteenth-century French dispute on the
nature of women and marriage (Bakhtin, 1968: 239 ff.). Here he
identifies contradictions in 'the Gallic tradition' with regard to
women between a profoundly negative Christian attitude, and the
exaltation of womanhood in 'chivalry':

> the Gallic tradition is a complex and contradictory phenome-
> non . . . it represented . . . two lines of thought: the popular
> comic tradition; and the ascetic tendency of medieval
> Christianity, which saw in woman the incarnation of sin, the
> temptation of the flesh.
>
> (ibid.: 240)

Bakhtin argues that these opposing views of women, although
frequently found intertwined, should be analytically separated as
they are, in fact, 'profoundly alien to each other' (ibid.: 240). The
unadulterated popular view of women is, he argues, neither
hostile nor negative, but celebrates women as part of the material
world:

woman is essentially related to the material bodily lower stratum; she is the incarnation of this stratum that degrades and regenerates simultaneously. She is ambivalent. She debases, brings down to earth, lends a bodily substance to things, and destroys; but, first of all, she is the principle that gives birth. She is the womb . . . the woman of Gallic tradition is the bodily grave of man. She represents in person the undoing of pretentiousness, of all that is finished, completed and exhausted.

(ibid.: 240)

It is, then, in the transition from the comic popular view to the serious ascetic view that 'ambivalence' becomes entirely negative. When the material realm as a whole is devalued as that which keeps the soul from heaven, women, as 'essentially related' to that realm, are devalued with it. But in true carnival imagery woman is the ultimate dialectical image: 'The woman's bowels are inexhaustible and never satisfied. She is organically hostile to all that is old . . . woman is naturally opposed to eternity' (ibid.: 242, 241).

A number of obvious points need to be made here. First, the *querelle* is, of course, a dispute between two masculine views of women, and we can have no idea what views women themselves held on the issue. Neither can we accurately gauge the participation of women in the generation of carnival imagery itself. However, I would suggest that the *querelle* does allow us a brief glimpse of differences in the conceptualizations of the male and female body in popular culture which the rest of Bakhtin's work unfortunately obscures (Booth, 1982; Miller, 1986). Here again, I would argue, gender difference is conceptualized as quantitative rather than qualitative. Women, as in the Christian view, are innately more material – more flesh than spirit.

While the distinction is similar, however, its effects are dramatically different. With the profoundly differing views of the 'degradation' of bodily life in popular and ascetic understandings, women's stronger connection with the material appears as strongly negative in the latter but positive in the former. In popular culture, as we have seen, the emphasis was on bodily openness and the fluidity of boundaries between the body and the world. The womb and the bowels are central images here, both acting to overturn and erase distinctions between body and world, life and death. Tentatively, then, we could accept Bakhtin's view that the popular notion of degradation as positive formed a 'pro-woman' strand in the socially dominant masculine view of women and the female body.

BOURGEOIS BODIES

Gurevich argues that in medieval categorizations people were part of nature, since 'the laws of creation are to be found in analogy' (Gurevich, 1985: 57). Consequently,

> the elements of the human body were identical, it was held, with the elements forming the universe. Man's flesh was of the earth, his blood of water, his breath of air and his warmth of fire.
>
> (ibid.: 57)

The unity of humanity and nature was experienced too in the feudal mode of production:

> Bound to the soil by his work, absorbed in the tasks of rural husbandry, man perceived nature as an integral part of himself instead of treating it as an object pure and simple to be manipulated, utilised or disposed of.
>
> (ibid.: 44)

Thus, as Gurevich argues, a 'subject–object' relationship between humanity and nature was impossible in feudal culture. The concept of human labour as 'transforming' nature was meaningless (ibid.: 54). For such a separation to be possible the 'distance' – both ideological and material – between humanity and the natural environment 'would have to increase' (ibid.: 67). This, of course, is precisely what happens with the transition to the capitalist mode of production, in which 'nature' *is* manipulable by human labour and can be transformed. As Gurevich argues:

> man's practical activity became more and more complex and his effect on nature more direct and purposeful, thanks to the development of new tools and the invention of machinery which came to adopt an intermediary position between man and his natural surroundings . . . he detaches himself more and more from her [nature] and begins to look upon her as an object to be utilised.
>
> (ibid.: 90)

Capitalist production separates humanity from nature, constructing nature as outside of the human subject, existing in order to be used. With the transition from feudal to bourgeois culture we see a transformation not only in the relationship of humanity to nature, but also in social relations. Power, wealth and status, previously vested in social role, seen as entailed in the fixed place occupied in a God-given hierarchy, come to be understood as the results of individual endeavour. Black and Coward argue that the modern bourgeois state:

> emerged in the disintegration of the relatively diffused hier-archy of the feudal state. Previously, political responsibilities and rights were derived from particular status given in a very definite hierarchy. The capitalist state, however, increasingly addressed its political representations to a generalized 'citizen' – sexless, classless, a citizen of the world.
>
> (Black and Coward, 1981: 83–4)

The notion of the generalized citizen is formed in the framework of capitalist social relations which depend on private ownership of the means of social production, and the justificatory ideology of possessive individualism. In feudalism, as we have seen, people are defined by their place in a rigidly hierarchical social order. In capitalism, 'free' labour and private ownership combine to create a social structure in which each worker is forced to sell her/his labour power as a commodity in competition with all other wor-kers, and in which each capitalist is in competition with all others in the rush to accumulate. Society is seen as the interaction of all these individual 'units' whose main motivation is self-interest, defined in terms of ownership. The change, as Bakhtin argues, is from the person as one element in the controlling hierarchy of the cosmos, to the perception of man (and I use the term advisedly) as the centre of the universe and its controller (Bakhtin, 1968: 366–7).

In bourgeois ideology the individual is king. Each individual acts in pursuit of his own interests; his social position is not fixed, but can with industrious effort be improved upon. Each individual is the agent of his own destiny, the centre of his universe. Conse-quent upon these material and ideological changes the concept of the body undergoes a transformation, in which separation and instrumentality characterize the bourgeois body. The chains that bound it to nature and to the collective body of the people having been broken, the body takes on a new meaning in the construction of nature as object and humanity as subject; it is used as an instrument in the pursuit of individual self-interest.

As we have seen, Bakhtin argues that the exaggerated bodily imagery of the medieval carnival reflects a collective understanding of the body as the body of the people. He contrasts this with modern ideas of the body as private, separate and individualized, 'the goal of egoistic lust and possession' (ibid.: 23, 19–24). The carnival focus on the parts of the body open to the world, and to the processes in which world and body intermingle is contrasted with the modern focus on the surface of the body as an impenetrable barrier between the individual and the environment (ibid.: 27, 39, 317–18). He argues:

> in the private sphere of isolated individuals the images of the bodily lower stratum preserve the element of negation while losing almost entirely their positive, regenerating force. Their link with life and with the cosmos is broken, they are narrowed down to naturalistic erotic images.
>
> (ibid.: 23)

The modern body is product rather than process – closed and completed, its links with the material degrading, in the modern sense, its imagery 'of the finished, completed man, cleansed, as it were, of all the scoriae of birth and death' (ibid.: 25, 24–6, 113). The individual body, then, loses its link with the material seen as a whole, in which it is not individualized but is rather 'a point of transition in a life eternally renewed, the inexhaustible vessel of death and conception' (ibid.: 318). In the popular medieval concept the body is irremediably a part of nature, and thus cannot be seen as an individual possession. The transition from feudalism to capitalism is in bodily terms the transition from the understanding of the body as a part and expression of nature, to the body as the vehicle through which the self expropriates and controls nature.

Bakhtin argues:

> the new bodily canon . . . presents an entirely finished, completed, strictly limited body, which is shown from the outside as something individual. That which protrudes, bulges, sprouts or branches off . . . is eliminated, hidden, or moderated. All orifices of the body are closed. The basis of the image is the individual, strictly limited mass, the impenetrable facade. The opaque surface and the body's 'valleys' acquire an essential

meaning as the border of a closed individuality that does not merge with other bodies and with the world.

(ibid.: 320)

The modern body is self-sufficient, an 'individual, closed sphere', and the focus of imagery is on 'individually characteristic and expressive parts of the body' – head, face, eyes, lips, muscular system (ibid.: 321).

Turner also takes up the separation of the body from its place in a fixed cosmology, and its transformation into an individualized possession with the emergence of capitalism. He argues:

the concept of nature as a world of physical objects independent of man and the concept of man as a thing-link phenomenon (a machine, an hydraulic pump, or as a cog within a clock) both emerged at a specific point in history, namely with the growth of commodity production within a fully monetarized economy.

(Turner, 1984: 232)

The emergence of the concept of the body as thing or commodity is further linked to the secularization of the body, in which the body is transformed from 'the object of a sacred discourse of the flesh' to the object of medical discourse which sees it as a 'machine to be controlled by appropriate scientific regimens' (ibid.: 36). Turner gives the example of Cheyne, who described the body as a hydraulic system the equilibrium of which is maintained by correct inputs and outputs (ibid.: 219).

Medical theory, Turner argues, was influenced in the seventeenth and eighteenth centuries by Descartes's privileging of the mind as the definition of the self. The body was simply a machine owned by the self, or person-as-mind, and medicine 'came to be markedly influenced by mathematical and chemical models of the body which was conceived as a complex machine' (ibid.: 77). For Hobbes the body was an 'extension' of the mind and he argued that man (as in man, not humanity) had 'a natural right to his own body' (and to the bodies of his wife and children) (quoted in ibid.: 87–9).

Capitalist conceptualizations of the body are, then, instrumental. The self uses the body as an individual possession. Turner pursues his argument through the changing concept of diet. As we have seen, in medieval asceticism dietary control was part of an attempt to control desire and to overcome the flesh. Turner argues that with capitalism desire/the body are fostered rather than

suppressed; the body must be disciplined in production but encouraged in its desires in consumption. This does not, however,
represent bodily 'freedom'; following Foucault, Turner argues
that desire is created and controlled through medicalized power,
and must thus be *correctly* channelled into consumption while
being controlled in production (ibid.: 159–70, 200).

Although desire and the body are created through and controlled by the legal and medical discourses of capitalism, they appear
as 'natural' and the 'suppression' of bodily desires at work and
their expression in the private sphere are seen as natural occur-
rences. The body, as a pre-given biological entity, and physical
desires, as naturally arising from biological dictates or 'needs', exist
a priori, to be used by the self as it chooses; the social construction
of the body and of desire are rendered invisible.

Diet is used in the twentieth century, Turner argues, 'in the
preservation of life to enhance the enjoyment of pleasures' (ibid.:
172). Consumption is a virtue rather than a sin, and 'diet is a
method of promoting the capacity for secular enjoyments': 'to be
complete persons we have to consume, to overspend and to satiate
desire' (ibid.: 216, 238). The body in consumer culture is, then, 'a
vehicle of pleasure' (ibid.: 172).

In this section two constructions of the bourgeois body will be
analysed in order to explore the argument that the body is constructed as fundamentally separate from, and acting upon, nature,
as private property, individualized and owned. Further, the construction of the body as gendered will form a central analytical link
between this and the following chapter. As Black and Coward
argue, the bourgeois concept of the individual citizen does not
include women (ibid.: 84). The subsequent argument seeks to
show that the concept of the individualized body, with its central
defining characteristics of separation and instrumentality, refers
not to the ungendered individual but to the masculine subject. The
feminine body, it will be argued, is constructed in oppostion to the
individualized body – as merged, rather than separate, and as
acted on, rather than active.

Victorian bodies

Barker-Benfield analyses the nineteenth-century perception of
the male body as a pseudo-economic system – 'the spermatic
economy'. The male body was seen as a self-sufficient system of

energies held in balance by reason (Barker-Benfield, 1976; 1973: 378). Its energies should be accumulated and disciplined, expended only in production – either of wealth or of babies – and any other expenditure was wasteful. The proper aim of a man was to 'discipline and utilise' his own bodily powers under the 'potent sway' of his mind (1973: 386, 380). He argues that: 'in working toward success one should conserve one's energies: having attained it, one had to be eternally vigilant to avoid debilitating expenditure' (1976: 296).

Work, then, used up physical energy, and the only other proper use for it was child production – the 'natural destiny' of sperm (ibid.: 267). He argues that the language of expenditure in nineteenth century masturbation phobia reveals 'an economy of the body' in which the masculine body was 'an economic system, whose fundamental orientation was the accumulation of resources': 'the underlying model for the operation of the whole man, psychological and physiological, was economic' (ibid.: 169, 195; 1973: 374).

The wasteful expenditure of sperm in masturbation or 'excessive' – i.e. non-procreative – sex, both of which were the subject of major public and medical concern in the second half of the century, 'drained the physical vigor otherwise available to the will', and first diverted and then removed men from the pursuit of success (1976: 176, 234, 171). Energy, like capital, should be 'developed, restrained, governed, not abrogated, destroyed, unrecognized' (ibid.: 235).

The masculine bodily economy was naturally self-sufficient – excessive 'drainage' of sperm upset its 'autonomous accumulation of energy' (ibid.: 178–9). Amariah Brigham explained the system:

> a fundamental law of the distribution of vital powers . . .[is] that when they are increased in one part they are diminished in all the rest of the living economy . . . to increase the powers of one organ it is absolutely necessary that they should be diminished in all the others.
>
> (quoted in Barker-Benfield, 1973: 375–6)

The proper aim of man was 'the hoarding and concentration of energy . . . in an obsessively self-sufficient system' (ibid.: 377). Spermatic expenditure should be productive, and there was much discussion on exactly how much intercourse could safely be seen as productive. The 'expenditure' of sperm should take place only under the guiding principles of the spermatic economy (1976: 181).

The rules could be quantified. Barker-Benfield discusses the anonymous author of 'Nocturnal emissions', writing in the *American Journal of Psychology* in January 1904:

> From 1895 to 1903 he calculated that he averaged 3.43 nocturnal emissions each month. Since he was a bachelor and did not masturbate, he felt that this was an accurate measure of permissable expenditures, and while 3.43 would vary for different men, it did represent the physiological limit that should be a warning to both 'unmarried masturbator and married incontinent'. His article is complete with statistics and a graph.
>
> (1973: 397)

Intercourse in the sunshine was also recommended, so that 'the copulators would be recharging their batteries even as they were discharging' (1976: 297–8).

We can see, then, how the necessity to accumulate capital and prioritize production over consumption in 'high bourgeois' culture provided the framework of social meanings through which the masculine body was conceptualized as a spermatic economy. Further, each bodily system is a strictly individual unit – each man must conserve and accumulate his own energy/capital in a body which is fundamentally self-sufficient. The mind must discipline and control the body in order that its energies can be used in production and accumulation. Bodily energies were men's constant capital; they were owned as absolute possessions, and were to be directed to work and the public sphere. The body was the vehicle through which reason acted on the environment.

To boldly go . . . . : gynaecologists as pioneers

In *The Horrors of the Half-known Life*, Barker-Benfield argues that the nineteenth-century view of women was of creatures simultaneously more like the angels and 'naturally closer to the animal' (1976: 85; 1973: 382). The two ideas coexisted in a 'dual view' of women. One ideological strand argued that women were innately sexually uninterested and delicately shrank from sex; the other saw women as dominated by the body, especially by the womb and the sexual appetites, to the extent that if not strictly controlled these appetites could 'extinguish' men and the social order.[2]

Feminists have argued that this dual view was expressed by women in hysterical symptoms – from the fainting fit or 'swoon' to the violent fit or 'paroxysm' – as well as in explanations for hysteria (see e.g. Smith-Rosenberg, 1972; Ehrenreich and English, 1973; 1979; Skultans, 1979; Showalter, 1981). The swoon was thought to be caused by the sexual repression which resulted from women's natural delicacy. On the other hand, however, Ehrenreich and English discuss tales of the sexually voracious hysterical women who made unseemly advances to impressionable young doctors in the privacy of medical consultation (Ehrenreich and English, 1973: 36).

Both ideological strands motivated the gynaecological surgery of the second half of the nineteenth century, and Barker-Benfield argues that this surgery must be seen as part of 'a defensive, emergency ideology' in the face of the first wave of modern feminism with its pressure for female education and reproductive control (Barker-Benfield, 1976: 84, 239). Gynaecology here, he suggests, functions as social control: 'the assertion of male supremacy seems to have been a response to fears of female encroachment' (ibid.: 87).

From 1870 onwards, Barker-Benfield argues, America witnessed 'a spate of gynaecological activity . . . characterised by flamboyant, drastic, risky and instant use of the knife'. Britain followed the same pattern, albeit 'more cautiously' (ibid.: 90; 1973: 382–3). Gynaecological journals, professional organizations, explanatory theories and the invention of new surgical instruments and techniques all flourished. Surgical treatment of the 'psychological' disorders of women was central in this expansion, and Barker-Benfield argues that 'the most spectacularly revealing of these surgical techniques were excision of the clitoris . . . and female castration' (1976: 89).

One of the most important figures in the new science of gynaecological surgery was J. Marion Sims, the inventor of the speculum. Sims's aim was to facilitate reproduction, and in this aim he believed himself hampered both by women's natural lack of sexual interest and the recalcitrant interior of her body (ibid.: 111, 116). He aimed to effect by surgery the sexual and physical openness which reproduction needed, and to which women, he believed, were naturally inimical. Sims also brought to medical attention and named the condition 'vaginismus' – spasmodic and involuntary contraction of the vagina (ibid.: 113). His cure for his

new condition was to anaesthetize the woman before intercourse
– in one case two or three times weekly for a year. Other 'Sims
specials' included hymen removal, incisions of the vaginal orifice
followed by dilation with wedges and incision of the cervix to
'facilitate' the passage of sperm and menstrual blood (ibid.: 114).

The theoretical background to his surgical work was the perception of female reproductive organs as resistant to impregnation;
one of his theories postulated 'a kind of spermatic rebound from
a recalcitrant canal wall' (ibid.: 112). Barker-Benfield argues that
Sims 'could not construe therapeutic action apart from preparing
women for pregnancy': Sims contrasted 'the sterile unimpreg-
nated uterus' with his 'ideal womb' – 'open to impregnation . . .
[having] a gagging, graceful form' (ibid.: 111, 113).

It was the speculum which made Sims's reputation; as Barker-
Benfield puts it, 'Sims raised himself from obscurity to the dazzle
of success by the elevation of women's organs from darkness into
the light' (ibid.: 94). Speaking of his invention, Sims presented
himself as an intrepid pioneer: 'I felt like an explorer in medicine
who first views a new and important territory' (ibid.: 95). Sims,
then, opened to masculine penetration by eye, speculum and penis
the hitherto mysterious feminine interior; Barker-Benfield suggests that Sims saw himself as Columbus, the vagina as his New
World (ibid.: 95).

If women's sex*less*ness legitimated this brand of surgery, it was
the opposite ideology of feminine voraciousness which legitimized
clitoridectomy and female castration. Clitoridectomy, invented in
the West as a surgical technique by the English gynaecologist Isaac
Baker Brown, at first coexisted with and was then superseded by
castration (in turn overtaken by hysterectomy). The first recorded
castration took place in 1872, and from 1880 until the turn of the
century the operation flourished (Barker-Benfield, 1973: 389).
Although it became markedly less common thereafter, women
were still castrated for psychological disorders as late as 1946
(1976: 121).

The aim of both castration and clitoridectomy was to make
'rebellious' women domestic and demure. The operation was used
to counter an increase – real or imaginary – in female masturbation, 'an activity which men feared inevitably aroused women's
naturally boundless but usually repressed appetite for men' (ibid.:
120–1, 122). Barker-Benfield argues that male gynaecologists
'without exception' were deeply concerned with feminine sexual

appetite; even those who opposed wholesale castration agreed it should be used on women 'manifesting uncontrollable desire' (ibid.: 125; 1973: 388). Gynaecologists 'tested' women 'for indications of the disease of desire by inducing orgasm, manipulating clitoris or breasts', and presented sexual surgery as an aid to feminine self-control, and the preservation of feminine fertility as a 'nationally-owned resource' (1976: 126, 132).

Underlying nineteenth-century sexual surgery, then, we can see a perception of feminine sexuality as potentially overwhelming and of the feminine body as dangerous to men. In *The Young Man* and *The Student's Manual*, the Rev. John Todd's popular and much reprinted anti-masturbation tracts, he describes a young man visiting a brothel as 'entering the door of woman whose house is the gate-way of hell' (quoted in ibid.: 171). Barker-Benfield argues that this image was intended to suggest entering the vagina in intercourse: 'Todd perhaps used a common image – hot, deadly and ubiquitous holes – for both masturbation and illicit sexual intercourse' (ibid.: 171). Here the feminine body is understood as draining masculine active energies. Women's uncurbed appetites, as well as masturbation, could keep men from production, success and wealth. Ejaculation weakened men; both in masturbation and in intercourse with women, with their 'sperm-sucking propensities' (ibid.: 131). The open genitals of women threatened the 'closed self-sufficiency' of men (ibid.: 128). The common association of sperm and money was mirrored in the sexual overtones of women's financial incontinence:

> Todd suggested her spending action was insatiable, and that she absorbed man's earnings, man's heart's blood, into her own absorbing system; her spending was 'the horse-leech which continually cries, Give, give, and which never says enough'.
>
> (ibid.: 194)

In the sexual and the financial sphere, then, woman could 'drain' men of sperm and money, through her 'interiorized draining power', her 'insatiable absorbtiveness', her 'bloodsucking' nature (ibid.: 195–6; 1973: 378, 381). The vagina and the womb were both seen as 'a consuming mouth', and 'the food it demanded was sperm' (1976: 271). The only way to effectively contain women's sexual appetites outside of surgery was to give them a *little* of what they wanted (1973: 379).

The medicalized social control of women sought to contain her dangerous body and sexuality and return her to her proper status as a 'reproductive machine', an 'inexhaustible and undemanding resource' (1976: 305, 198; 1973: 383). Barker-Benfield concludes that the aim of this control was for men to 'assimilate women's power to themselves just as they attempted to do with the rest of the resources of the earth': women's bodies and nature's body should both be subject to masculine mastery (1976: 202; 1973: 382, 391).

It is clear, then, that the contradictory notions of women as passive domestic beings naturally 'shrinking' from sex, *and* as insatiable 'drainers' of masculine sexual energies coexisted in Victorian ideology. The purity of womanhood, argued to be natural and innate, seemed to require a vast network of legal, medical and ideological controls to maintain it, controls which acted to contain the shadow-image of the delicate female, the insatiable woman. Barker-Benfield argues thus:

> So underlying men's wish that their women be delicate, not sensuous, even frigid, was the apprehension that women were by definition always on the verge of being sexually appetitive . . . a woman's physical capacity for sexual intercourse was un-limited, in direct contrast to a man's.
>
> (1976: 276–7)

The suppressed and contained power of women and of women's bodies was felt to be dangerously powerful and threatening to men; uncontrolled, women became 'all appetite', their bodies transformed from passive vessel to pump, a dark, hot and open space which perpetually threatened to engulf and extinguish the self-contained masculine body and patriarchal order itself (1973: 384, 374, 293). Men's bodies were spermatic economies; women's bodies were simultaneously the terrain of productive labour and of an uncontrolled consumption which threatened to swallow up the stockpiled energy of man.

Twentieth-century bodies

Sociobiological explanations define the twentieth-century body. Here, the body is presented as a purely biological organism, and the aim of discussion is to determine how organic/biological properties, seen as innate and natural, affect social life and human behaviour. Sociobiology explains the body as an individual possession which is the basis of biological accumulation, with sperm and egg representing the constant capital on which that accumulation is based.

Such sociobiologists as Trivers and Dawkins, following the work of the biologist W. D. Hamilton, argue that the motivating force behind human behaviour is the pursuit of individual genetic self-interest: the aim is to maximize the reproduction of our 'own' genes. Women, they argue, 'invest' more biological matter in an egg than men do in sperm and thus naturally immerse themselves in chastity and childcare; men, on the other hand, seek to impregnate as many women as possible, without being trapped into childcare and sexual faithfulness (see Sahlins, 1977: 4; Sayers, 1982: 51–3). Competition, male promiscuity, female faithfulness and male aggression are all 'explained' in this handy system.

There are, of course, a number of problems with this thesis, as Sayers and Sahlins point out (Sahlins, 1977; Sayers, 1982). Even if we accept the theory on its own terms, we might well ask whether the loss of male reproductive fitness in the competition for females, plus the weakening of women's position by male mass abandonment might not be counterproductive to individual genetic interests. Further, anthropological evidence amply demonstrates that the gender roles of chaste female and promiscuous male which sociobiology argues are direct products of biology are far from universal. If we accept that 'innate' biological drives shape human social institutions, how do we explain cultural diversity and historical change in human societies?

For present purposes, however, it is the fundamental circularity of sociobiological arguments which are relevant. Sociobiological theories rely on *social* presuppositions: it is only within a system based on private property that certainty of paternity is necessary – in order to pass on property; and it is only within a free labour system that trying to secure help with childcare would be either possible or necessary. Sociobiological explanations of human behaviour naturalize existing social relations, maintain privilege, and thus operate as social control. As the BSSRS Sociobiology Group point out: 'because most of them [sociobiological arguments] provide a "natural" explanation for the existence of social practices that appear unjust, they can be used to justify the practice' (1984: 132).

Sociobiological theory is, however, a crude theory on which to practise the skills of sociological critique. The ideology of the body

as individual possession reappears, however, in much more sophisticated analyses. Turner, as we have seen, isolates the notion of
'embodiment', which he defines as our direct sensual experience
of our bodies and argues that it is our sense of embodiment or
'corporeal government' which is the basis of individuality (Turner,
1984: 251). In a thoroughgoing sociological view of the body this
line of reasoning is problematic; why do we except 'individual'
sensual experience, or embodiment, from culture?

In *The Problem of Embodiment* Richard Zaner analyses Marcel's,
Sartre's and Merleau-Ponty's theories of embodiment. He argues
that consciousness is only possible as a result of embodiment, and
that the body only becomes animate organism rather than mere
physical matter through consciousness's 'intentiveness to it *as* its
own animate organism' (Zaner, 1971: viii, vii). Zaner seeks to
distance this understanding from Cartesian dualism, or the
'mind/body problem' in which the mind is seen to exist 'in' the
body – he argues that consciousness is embodied 'by' rather than
'in' the physical body (ibid.: vii). He suggests that his three chosen
writers attempt to 'overcome', or 'undercut' simple mind/body
dualism by addressing the problem Descartes himself recognized,
and which led to the original opposition of mind and body:

> the peculiar circumstance that, though my mind is not like my
> body, nor my body like my mind, nevertheless I am not 'in' my
> body like a boatman is 'in' his boat.
>
> (ibid.: 240)

We act *through* the body; it is the 'means of having a world and of
acting within it' (ibid.: 240). Objects in the world, including other
people, only exist meaningfully as objects which have a relation to
the person-in-the-body:

> objects in the world, in so far as they *are* for me only in virtue of
> my being embodied in the midst of them by my body-proper,
> and are thus disclosed as essentially connected to my possible
> bodily action on and with them.
>
> (ibid.: 240)

Mechanical conceptions of the body as matter animated and
owned by a mind conceived of as separate from that body are here
undermined. To what extent, however, do such arguments affect
the concept of the body as individualized possession?

One could argue that philosophizing at this level has effected common-sense understandings very little. The fine distinction between *having* and *being* in a body is not widely understood. Further, while Zaner's argument does undercut the very crude mind/body dualisms of, for example, Cheyne, it remains dualistic itself in its distinction of mind and body. Finally, the individuality of embodiment is unquestioned: the perception of the body is of an object separate from the world and acting upon it.

This issue is also present in the psychological concept of 'separation/individuation', as we saw in Chapters 2 and 3. Here the notion of the self and the body as separate – first, from the mother – is argued to develop as the infant begins to perceive itself/its body as having boundaries which distinguish it from the environment. This process develops through the baby's gradual perception that food/the breast is given and taken away, and thus is not part of itself. This process gradually extends so that the infant understands her/himself to be an individual entity or subject distinguished from the world of objects, and with desires to appropriate or act on that world of objects which originate within the self and the body.

In this view, as Parveen Adams points out, the body is constructed through libidinal desires (Adams, 1986: 29). The development of a 'secure' identity as an individual depends on the construction of a sense of the self and the body as separate from the world – having strong 'ego-boundaries' – and in the ability of the self to act upon the separated world of objects in order to fulfil desires and needs which arise *within* the self and the body.

An example of how the integrated self is held to develop can be found in the work of Melanie Klein (Klein, 1975). As Janet Sayers points out, Klein argues that the fear of annihilation is the infant's primary anxiety, and that this arises from the 'death instinct'. When the child's wishes – for food, or for comfort – are frustrated by the mother, the child's sense of itself as integrated or whole is so unformed that it cannot distinguish the object of that frustration (the mother) from itself, and thus fears that it will be destroyed by its own frustration. The defence against this anxiety is projection, through which the mother is seen as the attacker. Sayers explains:

> This gives rise to persecutory anxiety ... against which the baby defends itself by splitting off and denying its experience of the mother as frustrating and persecuting. Instead it idealizes her

as totally good, loving and gratifying – in sum, as the very
embodiment of the Life instinct.

(Sayers, 1987: 28)

This situation, however, should be temporary. Klein argued that
integration is an innate human tendency, in which life and death
instincts increasingly fuse, and a sense of the self and the mother
as whole and separate, containing both good/loved and bad/hated
elements is constructed. As the sense of the self as whole develops,
the confidence that the self contains within it the possibilities for
fulfilling its own needs develops, and the self is constructed as
independent and able to control its own life without dependence
on an all-powerful other (ibid.: 28–30).

Orbach and Eichenbaum also adopt a perspective in which
separation/individuation is seen as the crucial step in the development of a healthy personality. They argue that:

The first two years of life are the most important time for the
development of the inner core of the person, the psyche and the
personality together . . . the ego . . . Part of the appropriate
empathy and nurturance is the ability of the caregiver to provide a structure, a containment, and a sense of boundaries for
the baby . . . Because the baby is in the process of developing a
sense of self and does not yet have any boundaries, the mother
must bring the boundaries into the relationship; she must relate
to the baby as a separate person . . . When secure ego development occurs, we see the baby beginning to maintain a sense of
self even when its caregiver is not present.

(Orbach and Eichenbaum, 1983: 14–16)

Developing boundaries, then, depends on a proper response to
needs by the caregiver/mother. This shows the infant that (inner)
needs can be met through the (outer) environment which is
essentially benign. If needs are not met consistently, psychological
separation is hindered since the infant is still 'yearning' and has
no secure sense that its needs will be met (ibid.: 17). Proper
development, however, gives 'a sense of wholeness' and 'authentic
experience of selfhood' (ibid.: 197). Maturity thus depends on a
secure sense of the self and the body as separate from the environment, or world of objects, and as capable of fulfilling needs and
desires through the manipulation of that environment. This is the
result rather than precondition of development; however, its

acquisition is to be expected, all being well, as the result of a normal upbringing.

Such discussions show what is and what is not to be questioned when talking about the body. We can argue about *how* consciousness and matter, mind and body relate, but both mind and body remain individualized and separate; Zaner argues:

> This quest, then, in each of their [Marcel, Sartre and Merleau-Ponty] works turns toward subjectivity, or consciousness, or, as with Marcel, the human self. And here we have seen that each of them is struck by a peculiar characteristic of human being, one so fundamental that for each it is considered the very essence of human reality: for man, *to be* is always and essentially *to be aware of himself* as such, to be able to withdraw into himself and put himself into question.
>
> (Zaner, 1971: 242)

Consciousness is fundamentally and naturally *self*-consciousness; the body is fundamentally and naturally *my* body. The body is a synthesis rather than a pre-existing unity, since the variety of ways through which we perceive the world – sight, touch, taste – are automatically united into the body-as-a-whole as the centre of perception (ibid.: 254–5). 'I' am the centre of experience, not one element in the structure of the cosmos, or part of the collective body of the people: 'My body, as Sartre stresses, is the orientational centre, O, in terms of which the world and its multiple objects are structured and organised' (ibid.: 250). Perceiving the self/body as the centre of the universe depends not on social structure and ideology but on the phenomenological given that we experience our own body uniquely – and differently from our perception of all other objects – from within (ibid.: 249, 259).

Theorizations which try to distinguish the body as the owned matter of the mind and the mind as existing 'in' the body should not be seen as rejections of the idea of the body as a possession. Rather, they argue about *how* the body is owned – not about whether 'ownership' exists at all. The body remains the vehicle through which consciousness/mind/self acts on an environment conceived of as fundamentally separate from it, although that separation is constructed in psychological development rather than existing a priori. And this physical and psychical individualism is seen as the basis of the development of the normal personality.

Similarly, although the theory of the unconscious *can* be used, as Lacan does, to challenge the dominant conception of the subject as 'a unified self-present subject, an "I" who exists unproblematically in and for itself' (Burniston *et al.*, 1978: 114) it is more commonly used to complexify but substantially maintain that conception, in arguing that an imposed unity, or integration of separate 'parts' of the self – conscious and unconscious, Life and Death instincts – will occur *naturally*.

Here I would argue, as Turner does, that the body is both 'natural' and 'cultural': it exists as a biological phenomenon the perception of which is only possible through social categorizations, and as 'natural' in Marx's sense in which nature is continually transformed through human social labour, the 'natural' limits on which are themselves transformed through the labour process. Thus the body as alive – or as 'animated organism', places its own strictures on its incorporation into the ideology of possessive individualism, in that seeing it as a commodity like all others is always open to problematization. As Brown and Adams point out, 'possession' of the body cannot entail its total control (Brown and Adams, 1979: 47).

Our understandings of the body are irremediably *social*, and represent an articulation of what exists and how we understand it. This seems to me to be essentially Turner's position, but I would question his distinction between the concept of embodiment of 'phenomenological' individuality and individuality as a social institution. This distinction must always be *analytical* – it does not exist a priori.

In short, what I am questioning is whether it is part of 'human nature' to perceive the body as individualized. I have suggested that the very different medieval concepts of the body provide some evidence that it is not, and in the next chapter I will argue that the modern concept of the feminine body further undercuts individualism-as-nature arguments by constructing the feminine body as part of the environment on which the masculine separated subject acts.

At this point, however, I would argue that we can identify the dominant bourgeois body-concept as that of an individualized and completed possession of the self which is finished (in normal circumstances) after the integration and separation of the formative years of infancy, and through which we pursue pleasure and satisfy our (internal) desires in the expropriation of the separated environment. As we saw in Part I, desires form the 'core' of the person. The autonomous pursuit of individual interests is, then, the model for both the body and the self.

The fit body: vehicle or environment?

The concept of the body at the centre of the 'fitness boom' of the 1980s and 1990s also engages with the understanding of the body as the vehicle for the pursuit of individual self-interest.

Fitness and health are big issues in comtemporary culture. Jogging, aerobics, anti-smoking/drinking/drugs campaigns and concern with chemical 'additives' in food all represent an increased concern with bodily health. Originally a middle-class phenomenon, the fitness boom has been taken up by capital, the mass media and the state, and its market is expanding. Turner calls such practices 'forms of secular asceticism' or 'calculating hedonism', and argues that anorexia is one of them (Turner, 1984: 201, 205). In 'body-maintenance' practices people are offered 'pseudo-liberation' through consumption – the body is disciplined in order to be able to consume more and consume better:

> the new hedonism . . . is not oppositional, being perfectly geared into the market requirements of advanced capitalism . . . hedonistic fascination with the body exists to enhance competitive performance. We jog, slim and sleep not for their intrinsic enjoyment, but to improve our chances at sex, work and longevity.
>
> (ibid.:112)

The healthy body is, then, 'the basis of the good life' (ibid.: 172). 'Healthy living', in the words of *Cosmopolitan* magazine, allows you to 'maximize your potential' (*Cosmopolitan*, September 1988). We become fit for consumption and have a positive *duty* to be fit:

> personal responsibility for health through exercise, diet and avoidance of drugs, reduces the tax-drain of curative medical intervention. There is consequently an alliance between the state, the medical profession and the healthy citizen. The monogamous jogger is the healthy citizen.
>
> (Turner, 1984: 221)

The social meanings and 'functions' of body-maintenance are, however, somewhat more complex. An increased concern with the body encapsulates two views of the body in ambiguous fashion. Further, the meaning of body-maintenance is gender-variable.

We can identify a concern to perfect the body-as-vehicle for consumption and individuation in body-maintenance strategies. If the body is fit the self can realize itself more efficiently – do more, enjoy more, produce more, consume more, in short, act on its environment more intensively and for longer, and this is the most commonly expressed rationale for fitness – to live longer and get more out of life.

However, body-maintenance strategies also encapsulate a sense of the body as the 'last resort' of a purely individual control of the environment. If we as individuals are relatively powerless to affect social structures we can at least control the environment of our bodies. This process can be characterized, as Herzlich argues in her work on illness and health as social constructions, as a move from an understanding of health as that which makes activity possible to health as an activity in itself (Herzlich, 1973). This process also represents a move from the body as the centre 'O' *from* which we act to the body as the locus *in which* we act, where the self acts on the body rather than on the world, living *in* rather than *through* the body.

Both meanings engage with the idea of human agency. As capitalist production eats further and further into 'nature' as a limit on human activity, social life as a human creation 'emerges' more and more as an issue. We can see more clearly what Turner calls the human capacity for 'transformative labour' (Turner, 1984: 229). The obvious social power to control and alter the environment, however, sits uneasily with the bourgeois ideology of capitalist social relations as 'natural', that is, expressive of a fixed human nature which is biological/genetic in origin and thus outside of agency. On the level of the body, body-maintenance strategies express this contradiction in seeing the body simultaneously as the vehicle for expansive action/consumption and the only environment over which the individualized self can exert any meaningful control.

For women, further, the ideology of femininity modifies both these meanings. First, in bourgeois patriarchal culture the feminine body is constructed as the environment on which the masculine subject acts, as the acted-on rather than the actor, the consumed rather than the consumer. Women's arena for action is also limited to the private sphere. Thus, women's ambit of personal control is fundamentally constrained, and in this context control of the body takes a particular significance. Wendy Chapkis argues that 'the exercise of control over the body compensat[es] for a basic sense of a life out of control':

> The pursuit of beauty is also one of the few avenues to success over which a woman has some measure of personal control. You can mould your body much more easily than you can force access to the old-boy networks or get the job you want, the promotion you deserve, the salary you need, the recognition you are owed.
>
> (Chapkis, 1986: 12, 95)

Second, as Chapkis argues, fitness for women means being fit to be looked at rather than fit to act. She points out that:

> Clearly the appeal of Jane Fonda's *Workout*, Linda Evans's *Beauty and Exercise Book* and Raquel Welch's *Total Beauty and Fitness Program* lies in the promise that they can get you in shape . . . While muscles may be in, pretty clearly only certain kinds of muscles on certain kinds of recognizably feminine bodies are really acceptable. The model of the youthful and physically fit woman ultimately is not a symbol of power so much as it is a symbol of the beauty of feminine control over appetites and age . . . the final product should never suggest that the . . . woman on display is anything but inviting, available and welcoming.
>
> (ibid.: 9, 13, 51)

The feminine body is constructed as 'inviting, available and welcoming' in opposition to the masculine body as self-contained, active and invasive. The two body-concepts are interdependent; we cannot meaningfully discuss them apart. This chapter, however, has focused primarily on the masculine or individual body, discussing the feminine body as derivative of it. In the next chapter this focus is reversed, and the construction of the feminine body in bourgeois culture will take analytical centre stage.

Chapter 6

The feminine body

In the previous chapter I traced the broad changes in the dominant understanding of the body over the transition from feudalism to capitalism. I argued that the central conceptual shift was from the medieval understanding of the body as one element in a hierarchically interlinked cosmology to the bourgeois perception of the body as instrument, used by the self to act on an environment seen as fundamentally separate. The analysis of Bakhtin's writings was used to show that, and give an example of how, dominant ideas can be challenged, and I would like to reiterate here that I do not intend to suggest that dominant body-concepts are the *only* ideas with significant social currency. What I *would* argue is that alternative conceptualizations are constructed *in relation to* dominant concepts: the medieval carnival degradation of the powerful by subsumption into the material depends, I would argue, on an existing hierarchy of elite and mass, heaven and earth, superlunary and sub-lunary.

The task of this chapter is to analyse in more detail contemporary understandings of the female body. I will argue that masculine bodily *integrity* – or closure, separation – is constructed in relation to, and depends on the maintenance of feminine bodily *openness*; and that masculine bodily *instrumentality* is defined in relation to the construction of the feminine *body-as-environment*. I will argue that dominant (masculine) and subordinate (feminine) body-concepts are created through a set of *oppositions* – open/closed, active/passive, hard/soft, muscle/flesh – and that consequently resistance to or changes in one affects or undermines the other.

Here I am arguing that a further conceptual change in body-concepts brought about by the transition from feudalism to capitalism is a different relationship between male and female bodies. What I am suggesting is that in feudal understandings the gender difference is one of *quantity*: the bodies of men *and* women are understood as flesh in opposition to spirit, but women are more flesh than spirit, men more spirit than flesh. The radical splitting of the sexual division of labour which occurred with the transition from feudalism to capitalism (see e.g. Rowbotham, 1977; Hamilton, 1978) had, of course, resonances on the level of the body. With the stronger separation of male and female experience broadly along the lines of the public/private dichotomy, gender roles polarized and, in the realm of understandings of the body, flesh, sex and bodily functions became fundamentally *female*. In the ideology of the body the gender difference, then, becomes a difference of *quality*: woman as body, man as mind.

To pursue this argument I will attempt to approach the concept of the body in bourgeois culture through a feminist framework. While I argue that the transition sees a conceptual shift in the understanding of the body as gendered, I do not want to lose sight of the continuous thread of patriarchal ideology which underpins this shift – that is, the perception of women and the female body as a threat to male order – however that order is defined.

To return briefly to Turner, the notion of women as threat is, for him, central. He argues that the female body is the main challenge to property and power – it is what needs to be controlled. Consequently, the sociology of the body is, in essence, the sociology of the control of female sexuality (Turner, 1984: 37, 114). He points out that in patriarchal social orders women do not control their bodies, which, as 'productive bodies' are possessions: 'although women have a phenomenological possession of their bodies, they have rarely exercised full ownership' (ibid.: 120, 233, 57–8). In patriarchy, then, women experience their bodies 'as objects which are ruled externally' (ibid.: 233).

For Turner, however, the term 'patriarchy' has a strictly limited meaning. His argument is that patriarchy has dwindled into 'patrism'; since, with possessive individualism rights are given to *people* rather than to *fathers*, and since, with capitalism, household property loses its central importance to social stability, property rights in women, too, are weakened, losing their 'systematic legal and political backing' (ibid.: 155, 135–41). For Turner male property rights over women's bodies fits into this history of the decline of patriarchal power; feminism uses the ideology of possessive individualism against patriarchy and patriarchal property rights over women's bodies change, in response to this attack, from a real, material power into 'a defensive ideological reaction' (ibid.: 137, 248).

It will be one task of this chapter, then, through a detailed consideration of patriarchal property rights over the feminine body, its reproductive power and its sexuality, to try and put patriarchy – in the feminist sense – back into the argument, by arguing for the power of patriarchy materially *and* as ideology, and against Turner's extreme economic determinism.

Further, I will try and make a presence out of the second major absence of Turner's thesis – the masculine body. What I would suggest here is that equating the sociology of the body with the control of the female body alone is phallocentric; in presenting the female body as 'the issue' Turner naturalizes the male body as the unanalysed norm against which the 'abnormal' or different female is defined. In so doing, it is all too easy to lose sight of why and how feminist attacks on patriarchal concepts – including that of the feminine body – are resisted. If, as I have argued, the two concepts are defined in opposition to one another, feminist redefinitions threaten patriarchal power. The struggle over social constructions of the feminine body cannot be adequately understood unless the masculine body too is seen as a social construction. If the active male is constructed in opposition to the passive female, her struggle to become active threatens him. If the female body becomes the instrument of the feminine self, it is lost as an environment for the masculine self.

So in this chapter, through a consideration of femininity and the feminine body, I will be trying to show that the construction of gender difference should not be seen as the definition of female difference in relation to male normality, but as the creation of *two* genders defined through a set of oppositions. I hope then to raise masculinity as an issue every bit as 'social' and every bit as contentious as femininity.

FEMININE BODIES: THE FEMALE BODY IN BOURGEOIS CULTURE

In the rest of this chapter my aim is to make the gender division visible in the bourgeois body-concept through an examination of the *ownership* and the *representations* of the female body. Here the central argument will be that the concept of the body as the separated and owned instrument of the self is phallocentric, presenting as human an understanding based on gendered experience. Analysis of the perceptions and representations of the female body in bourgeois culture reveals a partially hidden subtext of the feminine body as unfinished, incomplete and potentially limitless. Further, this sub-text is intrinsically unstable, being understood simultaneously as a symbol of vulnerability and powerlessness on the one hand, and of voraciousness and threat on the other.

This sub-text is, however, hidden beneath a formal extension of the rights of the autonomous individual, beginning in the late nineteenth century, to women, and therefore of the concept of the individualized body to the female body. This obscurity can render invisible the continuing oppression of women, and places two fundamentally contradictory sets of expectations on women's shoulders: to be independent and separate while still remaining dependent and responsive. What I am suggesting is that for women there is a hidden and unresolvable tension in social expectations, and that this is expressed on the level of the body in the virgin/whore dichotomy, which feminists have long placed at the heart of the patriarchal control of women.

I will begin, then, by looking at patriarchal property rights in women's bodies through an analysis of the control of women's reproductive capabilities and sexuality. Here I will argue that the feminine body is understood as a marketable commodity, and as part of the environment on which the masculine subject acts.

I will then go on to look at the tensions between surface and interior in representations of the feminine body, analysing the flawless *exterior* of the ideology of beauty and the empty, voracious *interior* of pornography, and will conclude by arguing that the dichotomies of open/closed, virgin/whore, autonomy/dependence in the concept of the feminine body define women as objects in relation to the masculine subject, and as simultaneously representative of *weakness* and *threat*.

WINE, WOMEN AND SONG: THE FEMALE BODY AS PROPERTY

In contemporary patriarchies the male's de jure priority has recently been modified through the granting of divorce protection, citizenship, and property to women. Their chattel status continues in their loss of name, the obligation to adopt the husband's domicile, and the general legal assumption that marriage involves an exchange of the female's domestic service and (sexual) consortium in return for financial support.

(Millett, 1977: 34–5)

Kate Millett argues that the changes in patriarchy achieved by nineteenth-century Western feminism were reforming rather than revolutionary, attaining 'notable reform in the area of legislative and other civil rights' and attacking patriarchal society's 'most obvious abuses' but failing to 'penetrate deeply enough into . . . patriarchal ideology' (ibid.: 64).[1] The central ideological tenet of patriarchy – that the male equals 'the human norm, the subject and referent to which the female is "other" and "alien"' – reasserted itself after the feminist challenge (ibid.: 4, 85).

The patriarchal opposition of subject (masculine) and object (feminine) is the main axis of social meaning around which gendered bodies are constructed. Its continuing social salience surrounds women's 'ownership' of their bodies with ambiguity, and the 'second wave' of feminism this century has seen as central to women's oppression both the *definition* of women solely through the body and the *control* of women through patriarchal control of reproduction and sexuality. Adrienne Rich, for example, writes of 'the implacable political necessity for women to gain control of our bodies and our lives' (Rich, 1980: 221). And Rich further points out the hidden nature of women's bodily oppression, arguing that:

The understanding that male–female relationships have been founded on the status of the female as the property of the male, or of male-dominated institutions, continues to be difficult for both women and men.

(ibid.: 195)

This difficulty in understanding, I would argue, arises from the phallocentrism of the ideology of individualism, which offers women a spurious and supposedly gender-neutral individuality which is continually undercut by the ideology of femininity and its construction of the feminine as the responsive complement to the masculine-as-norm. I want to analyse these ambiguities by exploring the issues of abortion and rape, focusing on both the status of the feminine body as the passive environment through which patriarchal property rights are expressed and the hidden nature of the articulation of the discourses of individualism and femininity.

Abortion: a woman's right to choose?

Control of their fertility by women is a central issue in modern feminism. The campaign for reproductive autonomy was one of the resuscitated movement's initial demands, and was from the first couched in terms of women's right to control their own bodies. As *Shrew* of February 1971 explained:

> We demand that women have control over their bodies. We believe this is denied until we can decide whether to have children or not and when we have them. This requires free and available contraception and free abortion on demand.
>
> (quoted in Brunsdon, 1978: 21)

It is often popularly supposed that the 1967 Abortion Act gave British women abortion on demand, but in fact it did not, allowing only for termination of pregnancy with the permission of two doctors if the continuation of that pregnancy would endanger the woman's life or health. Abortion, while possible, is not, then, 'free on demand'. Women do not have the absolute right of disposal over the contents of their wombs, and this limits the extent to which women can be said to own or control their bodies. Further, abortion rights are by no means secure; there have been several attempts to limit access to abortion since 1967 in Britain, and Adrienne Rich writes of the American situation that abortion law is 'everywhere in jeopardy', threatening women with an 'elemental loss of control' over their bodies (Rich, 1980: 196). As Rosalind Pollack Petchesky argues, legal abortion in Britain and America 'hovers tenuously' in a patriarchal culture (Petchesky, 1986: vii).

Further, legality has ensured neither actual access to abortion or legitimation. As Lynne Segal points out, in spite of women's greater control of their fertility:

> we have yet to win the necessary feminist battle to establish women's right to choose to terminate an unwanted pregnancy: only 50 per cent of women now manage to obtain an NHS abortion, and this government has prevented research on a new

abortion pill which could be taken in the early weeks of pregnancy.

(Segal, 1987: 228; see also Oakley, 1987: 53)

The intense public debate over abortion has come to centre
around 'inalienable' rights: the 'right' of the foetus to life; the
'right' of women to have reproductive control; and occasionally
the 'rights' of men to 'have a say' in the decision to terminate a
pregnancy. Ellen Willis argues that this shift in focus represents 'a
psychological victory' for anti-abortionists. Writing in 1984, Willis
pointed out:

> Two years ago, abortion was almost always discussed in feminist
> terms – as a political issue affecting the condition of women.
> Since then, the grounds of the debate have shifted dramatically;
> more and more, the Right-to-Life movement has succeeded in
> getting the public and the media to see abortion as an abstract
> moral issue having solely to do with the rights of foetuses.
>
> (Willis, 1984a: 92)

This position, Willis points outs, rests on 'a crucial fallacy' – that
the rights of women and of foetuses can be isolated from each other
(ibid.: 92). Petchesky, too, argues that 'the symbolic fetus' and its
rights as *autonomous* from those of the pregnant woman, has
displaced women from the centre of the abortion debate (Petchesky, 1986: viii).

The rhetoric of rights, then, masks the *political* nature of the
struggle over reproduction. That the rights of the foetus are
presented as independent of women's struggle for control of their
bodies obscures the place of abortion in the power struggle over
women's 'productive bodies'; presenting 'foetal rights' as an abstract moral issue hides the question of *in whose interest* those
'rights' are advocated, and whose 'rights' they curtail.

Underlying that rhetoric lies a debate about the ownership and
control of women's sexuality and reproductive capacity which has
changed in focus from contraception to abortion as the political
struggle continues. Partial control of reproduction through contraception being substantially won in the West, women now seek
absolute control and public acknowledgement through the law of
that control. The object of reproductive control in contraception
is the unfertilized (in abortion, the fertilized) ovum – the evidence
that women's bodies are masculine territory. While women have

won control over their 'own' biological matter, ownership of the fertilized egg is seen as more contentious; in spite of the arguments from sociobiology that women's childcare responsibilities are the result of a much greater primary biological 'investment' in children, this greater investment does not automatically lead to greater rights – or ownership (see Gallagher, 1987).

Willis quotes from an interview with Ken Kesey, an anti-abortionist even in cases of rape: 'You don't plow under the corn because the seed was planted with a neighbour's shovel' (quoted in Willis, 1984a: 95–6). Women's bodies and reproductive capacities are, in the last instance, masculine property or, as Petchesky puts it, 'passive vessels' in reproduction (Petchesky, 1986: xv). She argues that in the abortion debate, as in the debate over new reproductive technologies, 'it is primarily the fetus, or embryo, which is the object of intervention'; the pregnant woman, 'whether as "donor" or "recipient", becomes merely the "site"' (ibid.: xvii). As Ann Oakley points out:

> The specific reproductive definition of women as mindless mothers appears to have emerged simultaneously with the move towards a centralized technological control of pregnancy which has taken place over the last thirty years . . . It has now become technologically possible to ignore the status of pregnant women as human beings.
>
> (Oakley, 1987: 39; see also Arditti, Duelli Klein and Minden, 1984; Corea, 1985)

Here Turner's argument that 'family' property becomes increasingly less important as property rights are lodged in individuals *as* individuals rather than as fathers is again relevant. However, even an acceptance of the argument that children as property become less important in a fully individualized society does not lead us to conclude that this is the only 'motive' for the patriarchal control of women. Patriarchal control of feminine sexuality as *responsive* is crucial here: women's struggle for autonomous control of reproduction can be read as a struggle over female sexuality, bodily control and ownership as a whole. I would argue that behind the rhetoric of foetal rights lies a struggle to control female sexuality. On the one side we find the struggle for abortion on demand, sexual freedom and physical autonomy, in which women claim complete rights of ownership in their bodies; on the other control through the ideology of foetal rights undermines that ownership.

As Willis argues, without abortion on demand, women who have not chosen to be pregnant face a loss of control over their lives and bodies; she writes:

> However gratifying pregnancy may be to a woman who desires it, for the unwilling it is literally an invasion . . . abortion is by normal standards an act of self-defence.
>
> (Willis, 1984a: 94)

The anti-abortionist response to this argument reveals, Willis argues, that 'the nitty-gritty in the abortion debate is not life but sex' (ibid.: 94). Pregnancy is seen as 'just punishment' for sexual activity – for women, that is; women have 'no right to selfish pleasure at the expense of the unborn' and must remain 'continually vulnerable to the invasion of their bodies' (ibid.: 94). The restriction of abortion, then, contains and controls female sexuality.

The abortion debate is one area in which the tension between individuality and femininity as social roles for women is expressed. As Petchesky argues, the ideology of individual rights is part of what keeps abortion legal – as the individual's 'freedom of choice' in an area of 'private morality' (Petchesky, 1986: ix). But if the formal consideration of women as individuals helps keep abortion legal, the sub-text of femininity continually undermines that 'individuality' by presenting women as masculine property, and threatens abortion rights.

Women are not fully 'individuals' in the abortion debate, but the foetus, ironically, is. Petchesky argues that images of the foetus suspended in amniotic fluid now so 'saturate' the debate that not even feminists question the distortion and decontextualization entailed in the presentation of a foetus 'as if dangling in space, without a woman's uterus and body and bloodstream to support it' (ibid.: x–xi).

Petchesky argues thus:

> Chaste silhouettes of the foetal form, or voyeuristic-necrophilist photographs of its remains, litter the background of any abortion talk. These still images float like spirits through the courtrooms, where lawyers argue that foetuses can claim tort liability; through the hospitals and clinics, where physicians welcome them as 'patients'; and in front of all the abortion clinics, legislative committees, bus terminals and other places

that 'right-to-lifers' haunt. The strategy of anti-abortionists [is] to make foetal personhood a self-fulfilling prophecy by making the foetus a *public presence*.

(Petchesky, 1987: 57–8)

The image, Petchesky argues, is neither, as is suggested by Dr Bernard Nathanson in the video entitled 'The Silent Scream', the view 'from the vantage point of the victim (fetus)' or the perception of the pregnant woman. Rather, it is the view of 'a male onlooker' (Petchesky, 1986: xi; 1987: 60–3). She quotes Barbara Katz Rothman:

> the fetus in utero has become a metaphor for 'man' in space, floating free, attached only by the umbilical cord to the space-ship. But where is the mother in that metaphor? She has become empty space.
>
> (Rothman, 1986: 114; quoted in Petchesky, 1986: xi)

Such imagery, and the rhetoric of the obstetric 'advances' which made it possible, eerily echoes the rhetoric and practice of nine-teenth-century gynaecological surgery which Barker-Benfield analyses. Petchesky argues that it presents the womb 'as a space to be conquered', and quotes from an interview with Bernard Na-thanson in *Newsweek*: 'With the aid of technology, we stripped away the walls of the abdomen and uterus and looked into the womb' (quoted in Petchesky, 1987: 69). Similarly Oakley argues that ultrasound acts as 'a window on the womb' (Oakley, 1987: 44). Dr Michael Harrison, discussing the use of ultrasound techniques, writes:

> The fetus could not be taken seriously as long as he remained a medical recluse in an opaque womb; and it was not until the last half of this century that the prying eye of the ultrasonagram . . . rendered the once opaque womb transparent, stripping the veil of mystery from the dark inner sanctum, and letting the light of scientific observation fall on the shy and secretive fetus.
>
> (quoted in Petchesky, 1987: 69)

Twentieth-century obstetrical technology, then, like nineteenth-century gynaecological surgery, allows masculine penetration of the 'dark inner sanctum' of the feminine body, and this penetra-tion, clearly, entails control. It allows, as Oakley points out: 'the treatment of women as objects, as biological systems manipulable in the interests of patriarchy, and only rarely themselves capable of manipulation' (Oakley, 1987: 51). Petchesky relates such imagery to 'the Hobbesian view of . . . human beings as disconnected, solitary individuals, paradoxically helpless and autonomous at the same time' (Petchesky, 1986: xi). Thus 'abstract individualism' embraces the foetus but blanks out the woman and the dependence of the foetus on her. I would argue, further, that it includes the symbolic *male* foetus in an individualism to which women do not have full access, suggesting that although entirely physically dependent the foetus and its 'rights' take priority over autonomous reproductive control for women. The foetus in this imagery, as Petchesky suggests: 'is not the image of a baby at all but of a tiny man, a homunculus'. The foetus is 'a "baby man", an autonomous, atomized mini-space hero' (Petchesky, 1987: 61, 64). The symbolic foetus, as masculine, is represented as 'primary and autonomous'; the pregnant woman, as feminine, is 'absent or peripheral' (ibid.: 62).

Women's bodies, then, are controlled as 'productive bodies' *and* as feminine bodies; the 'abstract individualism' (ibid.: 63) of the abortion debate seeks to prevent the autonomous sexual action of women as well as to control the 'products' of the female body.

Rape: the right to say no?

Feminists working in the area of sexual violence against women have long argued that the dominant legal and popular understandings of rape are seriously flawed. Feminists argue that rape, far from being the rare act of a psychopathic stranger, is in fact an extremely common act which takes to the 'extreme and logical conclusion' 'normal' heterosexual relations in which coercion is present to a greater or lesser degree in the majority of sexual encounters (LRCC, 1984: 5). Box, for example, argues that rape 'is not the opposite to normal sex but a grim, grinning caricature of it' (Box, 1983: 150) and Clark and Lewis argue that rape is the 'price' we pay for a coercive standard in heterosexual relations (Clark and Lewis, 1977). Rape, then, is one expression of a sexual politics in which patriarchal power is played out: it depends, for its meaning and existence, on unequal power relations which exist across the spectrum of the social relations of the genders. As Andrea Dworkin argues: 'men are a privileged gender class over and against women. One of their privileges is the right of rape –

that is, the right of carnal access to any woman' (Dworkin, 1982: 40).

Lynne Harvie argues that public abhorrence of the crime coexists with an underlying and widespread belief that much of the responsibility for rape can be found in the negligent or provocative behaviour of women. She suggests that public abhorrence is based on the stereotypical stranger-in-a-dark-alley rape which is, in fact, comparatively rare (Harvie, 1986: 1). In the majority of rapes which do not fit this stereotype much, if not all of the blame is placed on the woman attacked; the stereotype acts to distance rape from 'normal' heterosexual relations. Harvie argues: 'the basic premise is that "normal men" do not rape. Therefore if a woman is raped by an "ordinary man" then she herself must be to blame' (ibid.: 19).

Largely because of this, reporting rates are low – 8 per cent in Hall's survey – conviction rates are very low and sentences rarely approach the maximum possible in statute (Clark and Lewis, 1977: 57; Chambers and Miller, 1987; Hall, 1985). Rape is the only crime in which going to trial is a better option than pleading guilty; sentences at trial are considerably lower than sentences from guilty pleas – the reverse of what happens in other crimes – because rape trials give defence lawyers the opportunity to argue that the real explanation for the attack is to be found in the behaviour of the woman (Chambers and Miller, 1987).

Feminists argue, then, that rape in reality *and* as ideology acts as social control. Susan Griffin describes rape as a male protection racket (Griffin, 1971; 1979) and Jacqueline Dowd Hall compares the effect of rape on women with that of lynching on Black Americans in the earlier part of this century – 'an instrument of coercion intended to impress not only the immediate victim but all who saw or heard about the event'; both rape and lynching, she argues, serve the political function of 'psychological intimidation' (Hall, 1984: 341, 340; see also Clark and Lewis, 1977: 23; Brownmiller, 1978).

What does the debate over the meaning, extent and function of rape tell us about the construction of the feminine body? Legal discourse on rape – both statutory and in practice – reveals that sexual autonomy is not one of women's rights: women are the sexual property of men. Rape law, indeed, originated as an explicit property law, as Clark and Lewis point out:

Under Anglo-Saxon law rape, along with most other offences, was punished by orders to pay compensation and reparation. If a woman was raped, a sum was paid to either her husband or her father, depending on who still exercised rights of ownership over her, and the exact amount of compensation depended on the woman's economic position and her desirability as an object of an exclusive sexual relationship. The sum was not paid to the woman herself; it was paid to her father or husband because he was the person who was regarded as having been wronged by the act.

(Clark and Lewis, 1977: 115–16)

Rape, then, was initially an act of *trespass* on a woman's body as male property, and Clark and Lewis argue that it 'has not lost the shrouds of these historical origins' (ibid.: 116). Their study showed that there exists an informal and extra-legal distinction of women into 'rapable' and 'unrapable' categories; to be a 'credible' victim of rape women must be clearly dependent on one male 'owner-protector', being either 'virgins under the ownership and protection of their fathers, or chaste wives under the ownership and protection of their husbands' (ibid.: 117).[2] They argue that what this implies is that women are sexual property, their sexuality is owned by the man they are dependent on, and that the value of sexuality-as-commodity rests on its potential for *exclusive* ownership. Their study found that 'the primary determinants of police classification are variables which describe the victim – her age, her marital and occupational status, her emotional and physical condition when she reported the crime' (ibid.: 77, 117). Two comparable studies in Scotland – *Investigating Sexual Assault* and *Prosecuting Sexual Assault* – found exactly the same; it is the characteristics of the woman which form the main criteria on which the decision on whether to proceed, and the trial itself, hinges (Chambers and Miller, 1983; 1987). The central criterion here is the woman's 'past sexual history'; if she is, or can be argued to be, anything other than a virgin or a faithful wife her 'credibility' is significantly reduced. Clark and Lewis argue that in practice, if not in statute, decisions on women's value as sexual property lie at the heart of legal action on rape: 'in effect, the law is saying that some women can be raped and some women can't' (Clark and Lewis, 1977: 92; see also Griffin, 1971: 2).

As we saw, originally *all* women were treated as property. Clark and Lewis explain the modern distinction thus:

> Women who voluntarily give up that which makes them desirable as objects of an exclusive sexual relationship are seen as 'common property', to be appropriated without penalty for the use, however temporary, of any man who desires their services . . . the voluntary granting of sexual access outside the parameters of sanctified matrimony leads to the loss of sexual and physical autonomy. Once a woman parts with her one and only treasure, she never has the right to say no again.
>
> (ibid.: 121)

Clark and Lewis argue that women who live outside of marital monogamy can be described as 'fair game', or 'open-territory victims' (ibid.: 123, 94). Rape law is still in essence property law, and does not provide women 'any guaranteed right to sexual autonomy' (ibid.: 124). As Griffin argues: 'One begins to suspect that it is the behaviour of the fallen woman, not that of the male, that civilization aims to control' (Griffin, 1971: 4). Until recently, the law in England and Wales stated that husbands could not rape their wives, since marriage represents continuous and irrevocable consent to sexual intercourse. Having once consented to intercourse with her husband a woman has no legal right to withdraw that consent. As Sally Vincent argues: 'A man cannot rape his wife because he cannot steal what he already owns' (Vincent, 1984; see also Dworkin, 1982: 29). While there is now a precedent that rape *can* occur in marriage, the few prosecutions which have been brought have all been in situations where the couple are separated. It will be interesting to see if, in practice, the concept of a husband's right to sexual access to his wife while she is living with him can be upheld within this new interpretation of statute.

This situation is mirrored in the 'extra-legal' standards of common sense and legal practice which imply that once a woman has willingly had extra-marital sex she is unlikely ever to refuse sex again – and has little real right to. In *Investigating Sexual Assault* Chambers and Miller quote from police case notes on rapes which were reported but not proceeded with:

> This self-admitted whore came out of a close at about midnight

and hailed two passing beat cops and told them she had been raped.

> She had had sex on a number of occasions in the past [and was] a bit of a loose female.
>
> (Chambers and Miller, 1983: 33, 42)

But if women do not have ownership rights over their sexuality, they do have *responsibilities*. Women are responsible for protecting the property, and preventing rape-as-trespass: Harvie argues that the police 'see a genuine rape as involving a high degree of physical violence and expect a woman to fight to the end to protect her honour'; she quotes one detective: 'she didn't resist to the last . . . then of course it's not rape' (Harvie, 1986: 20, 91). As well as physically resisting an attack, women are also expected to prevent it arising in the first place by 'unprovocative' dress and behaviour, by restricting their mobility and by not 'leading men on'. A Detective Sergeant interviewed by Chambers and Miller explains the argument:

> I think it's a crime [in] which a lot of young men . . . can find themselves genuinely raping someone . . . being overcome . . . led on to a certain point where there's no going back.
>
> (Chambers and Miller, 1983: 93)

Feminine sexuality, then, acts as a stimulus to masculine desire. Dominant discourses on rape imply: 'that it is women who cause rape by being unchaste or in the wrong place at the wrong time – in essence, by behaving as though they were free' (Griffin, 1971: 6). Women must police their sexuality in order to protect themselves from rape. As Griffin argues, women thus learn 'to distrust . . . [their] own carnality' (ibid.: 6). Women learn to fear their own sexuality and what its exercise may provoke. Once it has been aroused, the male sex-drive is seen as uncontrollable; responsibility for unleashing it lies with women (Harvie, 1986: 4).

Women, then, act as *caretakers* rather than owners of their bodies and their sexuality. As Clark and Lewis argue:

> Prior to marriage, a woman's sexuality is a commodity to be held in trust for its lawful owner. Making 'free' use of one's sexuality is like making 'free' use of someone else's money. One can act autonomously only with things that belong to oneself.
>
> (Clark and Lewis, 1977: 122)

Women do not have rights of disposal over their sexuality; while virginity is property held in trust, marital monogamy equals exclusive ownership. However, what cannot be bought can always be stolen. Dominant discourses on rape construct the feminine body as patriarchal property, and relate rape to women's sexual behaviour. This, I would argue, has three main effects. First, the identification of women's sexual behaviour as the true cause of rape alienates women from their sexual desires, which they must 'self-police'. Second, women are alienated from their bodies which are, in the last instance, the sexual property of others. In rape, feminine subjecthood is annihilated; women's bodies are directly treated as objects. Diana Russell, in her study of rape, quotes one of her interviewees:

> There's something worse about being raped than just being beaten. It's the final humiliation, the final showing you that you're worthless and that you're there to be used by whoever wants you.
>
> (Russell, 1975: 77)

As Griffin argues: 'Rape is an act of aggression in which the victim is denied her self-determination'; she becomes 'the object and not the subject of human behaviour. It is in this sense that a woman is deprived of the status of a human being. She is not free to be' (Griffin, 1971: 8, 6). Finally, the obligation to maintain a physical integrity of which virginity is the only true expression leads to a tension in the relationship of surface and interior. If physical integrity is to be maintained the body must be impregnable; if women wish to be heterosexually successful the body must yield.

In the next section the contradiction between bodily surface as impregnable and bodily interior as receptive will be explored, and we shall see how this tension interacts with the obligation on women to construct their bodies as attractive objects, as, in Stannard's term, 'articles of conspicuous consumption in the male market' (Stannard, 1971: 123).

SURFACE TENSION: SKIN AS SYMBOLIC VIRGINITY

'Virgins must be boring to go to bed with' said Chloe, looking directly at Simon. 'They don't know first base from second.'

'When I was a child I liked popping balloons, and fuschia buds,' said Simon softly. 'I always like putting my finger through the paper on the top of the Maxwell House jar. I like virgins. You can break them in how you like, before they have the time to learn any bad habits.'

(Jilly Cooper, 1977: 22–3)

Bakhtin, as we have seen, argues that the focus of the bourgeois body is the surface of the body as 'opaque' and 'impenetrable' facade, through which the body is understood as non-merging and totally individual (Bakhtin, 1968: 320). I have suggested that the presentation of this body-concept as gender-neutral is phallocentric, referring as it does to a dominant masculine 'text' and ignoring the feminine 'sub-text'. I would argue that this total bodily 'closure' is a *masculine* posssibility; however, this does not prevent closure being presented as a goal for women. Striving for closure is, however, undercut for women by their simultaneous duty to be open and receptive. Masculine separation and feminine openness are not, of course, equal in value. Receptivity is fundamentally ambiguous, and represents weakness, vulnerability, and, as we shall see, potential voraciousness. The articulation of separation and openness is a basic task of femininity; in feminine bodily self-discipline the articulation of impenetrability and receptivity is the central task.

The cosmetic exterior: 'There is this woman. Watch her'[3]

One expression of the tension between integrity and openness is the obsession with the surface of the body, with, in Bardwick and Douvan's term, 'the cosmetic exterior'. Women construct their bodies as attractive objects, as stimuli for masculine desire, and Bardwick and Douvan argue that the function of the cosmetic exterior is 'to lure men, to secure affection, to succeed in the competition of dating' (Bardwick and Douvan, 1971: 150–1).

Una Stannard in 'The mask of beauty', argues that:

Little girls look endlessly at beautiful women. They hear and read about them too . . . [the girl] compares herself to the media ideal of beauty and is usually found wanting. She then begins woman's frantic pursuit of beauty . . . in this culture women are told that they are the fair sex, but at the same time that their 'beauty' needs lifting, shaping, dying, painting, curling, padding.

(Stannard, 1971: 118–22)

Attractiveness is central to femininity, and is also a billion-dollar industry. The standards aimed at are never really achieved – an airbrushed and retouched studio image can never really be replicated, even if the raw material of the 5 foot 10, size 8, 17–year-old model were not a world away from the body of the average woman. Beauty is an unachievable ideal which fuels consumption; not only do women have to spend to maintain their looks, but there is always the possibility that the latest new product or 'scientific' cosmetic discovery will be the one to help them really achieve the unachievable. As Marjorie Ferguson points out in her study of women's magazines, the ideology of beauty 'presents the desirable as though it were possible': 'second only to messages of female obligation to maximise physical attractiveness are promises of its attainability' (Ferguson, 1983: 58; 59).

The construction of women's bodies as sexual objects is exploited and amplified by capitalism; the frantic pursuit of unattainable beauty and the frantic pursuit of profit walk hand in hand. The effects of this objectification have been well-documented by feminists. Ann Oakley, for example, argues that women experience alienation from their bodies, expressed in 'the careful watching of one's body and its fabrication as a public viewing object' (Oakley, 1981: 82; see also Chapkis, 1986). Women's bodies are 'on show'; they are obliged to produce their bodies as adequate and acceptable 'spectacles', as objects external to their selves.

Two meanings of the social obsession with female appearance are, then, obvious, and have become, to an extent, feminist clichés. Women's bodies provide a continually expanding market for capitalist production; women's bodies are the 'lure' which attracts male sexual interest. Women produce the cosmetic exterior as an object for men and for capital; the beauty obsession colludes with femininity, dependency and consumerism.

What I would like to go on to look at, however, are some more complex contradictions which the messages of the beauty industry reveal, and which, as we shall see, problematize the idea of the pursuit of beauty as simple passive acceptance of stereotypical femininity.

'Improve your outline': smooth, firm and tight

> With the pips of an apricot, women can slow down the seeds of
> time.
>
> (Kanebo Sensai Skincare)[4]

The cosmetic exterior functions both to attract and to discipline. While creating the body as beautiful is geared to attracting the interest and approval of men, it is also constructed as an exterior, a mask, a barrier.[5] If we look at beauty messages about female skin we can see that the dual aims are receptivity, expressed as softness, and closure, represented as 'flawlessness'. Women work on the skin as surface from the outside with make-up, cleansers, depilatories and surgery, and from the inside with diet and exercise; the aim of both processes resembles with remarkable exactitude Bakhtin's 'new bodily canon' – the opaque and impenetrable bodily surface, cloaked in the acceptable and expected feminine goal of being soft to the (masculine) touch.

The enemies of smoothness, firmness and tightness are legion – spots, wrinkles, veins, stretch marks, hard skin, dry skin, sweat, hair and flab. Fortunately, however, they can all be dealt with – with a little help, of course.

Preparation

> Skin looks lumpy, bumpy, dingy? Uneven in tone and texture? Don't panic – it's surprising what a daily dose of friction rubbing and a dollop of moisturiser can do to neglected skin. With a soapy loofah or friction sponge, scrub skin til it tingles, particularly the areas that get rough and 'goose-pimply' . . . a good scrub like this bucks up sluggish circulation and also gets rid of any dead surface cells, so skin not only feels instantly smoother but is all set for a smoother suntan too.'
>
> (Carol Grant, 1987)

There's a lot of work to be done before women put on their make-up. Although the focus is often on the face, the entire surface of the body must be worked on, made smooth and flawless. Louis Marcel's Smooth Operators range is produced in different packages for the whole body – extending right down to the feet: 'Remember feet? Those neglected things at the end of your legs?'

Moisturisers prevent dry skin's attack on the smooth surface;

exfoliators expunge the danger of 'dead surface cells'; Louis Marcel can eliminate hard skin from your feet; anti-perspirants keep you 'dry and silky', banishing sweat; depilatories help you 'say goodbye to fuzz' ; and Vichy helps you 'fight back at wrinkles – iron out surface lines – tighten up the skin'.

For women who need just that bit more, Biotherm and Chanel are waiting in the wings with a new range of 'scientific' products which will actually affect muscle 'tone': 'Chanel Lift Serum Antirides-Raffermissant' with 'Plastoderm' will 'gradually fill . . . out laughter lines and wrinkles . . . tone, tighten and smooth'. Biotherm's 'skin-firming range' hits all those problem areas with Exfoliating Body Scrub, Active Body Skin Firmer, Stomach Firming Treatment and 28-day Bust Firmer. And Clarins' Skin Firming Concentrate both identifies and solves 'the problem':

> Slackening skin? Be firm with your face . . . Throughout the day the highly effective, active ingredients will be working to tone and firm skin tissues, helping to smooth out fine lines, improve the texture of your skin, and restore firmer facial contours.

Approaching the same goal from the opposite angle, diet and exercise erradicate 'flab'; Carol Grant, skin evangelist, tells us how:

> Fight the flab. Spare tyre, flabby thighs, bulging tum? No miracles promised, but 20 minutes a day of exercises, combined with a quickie diet, will definitely improve your outline.
> (Grant, 1987; see also Coward, 1984: 40)

The surface has been primed; the next stage awaits.

Presentation

The basic principle of the cosmetic exterior is a smooth foundation – from this all else flows. *Woman* magazine explains:

> The purpose of foundation is to provide a better-looking skin, both in terms of colour and texture. The film it leaves on your skin hides minor blemishes and gives you colour too.
> (*Woman*, 5 Sept. 1987)

'Even' skin tone has two meanings: skin has to feel smooth (texture) and look smooth (colour). The aim of cosmetic labour is to look as though there has been no work done at all: 'Barbara Daly shows you how to create the perfect natural face . . . the face you can put on in the morning and stay happy with all day' (*Woman*, 5 Dec. 1987). Elizabeth Arden Simply Perfect Mousse Make-up 'gives you *incredible coverage* to even out skin tones . . . Result? A perfect, fine-textured finish that looks natural, glowing, fresh for hours.' Clinique Pore-minimizer Make-up can go even further; it's not just 'flaws' which disappear but pores too: 'Women wanted a make-up that gives any skin a flawless finish. One that makes pores seem to disappear.'

Repair

If all this still doesn't work, women can relinquish the 'natural' apricot seed for electronic technology and cosmetic surgery. If Plastoderm, exercise and diet can't tone and firm your skin, 'don't panic' – there's always Minitone:

> Minitone gets right down to the face-shaping muscles beneath the skin . . . the first effect you'll see is a gradual lifting and firming of the chinline. Then, as the facial muscles really start responding the lines around the mouth should begin to fade.

Or Speedshaper:

> Turn belly flab into a super flat stomach! Tummy muscles slack and out of shape? . . . you can discover the new method of trimming away ugly embarrassing flab . . . to reveal a brand-new firm, trim and shapely body.

Or the new portable Stomach Trimmer:

> Gives you a slim, trim stomach in just 5 to 10 minutes a day . . . Pull up – relax, pull up – relax, to tone and firm those muscles . . . whenever you've got a spare moment use it to trim that stomach down.

The function of muscle then, is not to move or to act, but to maintain the firm, taut outline – to 'keep it in' (see Coward, 1984: 21). And if do it yourself can't do it, there's always cosmetic surgery. Wrinkles can be 'filled out' by 'collagen' injections (*Sky* magazine, 21 Aug. 1987), and if that won't fit the bill you can always go the whole hog and have a face lift.

The perfect end product, then, is smooth, flawless, tight and firm – or, impenetrable, opaque and closed. As Ferguson points out, it is both sexual and asexual: 'It is sexual in defining the female state as pleasingly attractive . . . it is a-sexual in offering a polished, perfected, depilated, deodorised object' (Ferguson, 1983: 63). Its unattainability in reality provides the impetus for a continual proliferation of products, going progressively deeper into the body, and seems to impinge not at all on the energy devoted to its pursuit. *Real* female skin will always have 'flaws' – wrinkles cannot be kept at bay forever, pores can't really disappear, and under the make-up uneven skin tone lurks. The image, however, can and does remain everlastingly flawless, reaching its zenith in a recent Chanel make-up advert where the eyes and mouth, sporting the 'latest' colours, appear isolated on the white page – skin so perfect it has vanished altogether.

The perfected skin offers no way in; its boundaries are firm and clear – they do not yield. The perfected skin covers the body as a protective barrier, its image, its symbolic value to create the impenetrable facade of the bourgeois body for penetrable woman; the reality, however, real skin, wrinkled, flawed, fuzzed and sagging, haunts the facade like a spectre at the feast.

THE PASSIVE VESSEL? VIRGINS AND WHORES

However justified men may believe their social position to be, they are nonetheless aware, at some level, that women are oppressed and do not always accept their oppression willingly. Misogyny is caused by fear as well as resentment, and as the Orpheus legend tells us, many men fear women deeply. There is always a possibility that the submissive housewife may turn into a bacchante or Medea, or (according to a more modern legend), a 'castrating' female . . . Men's fear of women, and the misogyny it produces, rests on the awareness that women have good reason to seek revenge.

(Clark and Lewis, 1977: 139)

That men hate and fear women seems almost to be taken for granted by many feminists; discussion of misogyny, further, frequently raises the idea of female sexuality and the female body as a threatening environment for men (Greer, 1971; Dworkin, 1974; Millett, 1977). Susan Lipschitz, for example, argues that popular images of prostitutes relate to 'an unconscious image of a feared, evil and sexual woman' (Lipschitz, 1978: 56). Underlying ideologies of female sexual passivity, it is suggested, lie deep anxieties about the social control of a force which continually threatens disorder and chaos. Katherine Arnold argues that women 'are not seen as able or willing to control themselves. They are suspected of harbouring desires which are inimical to the smooth functioning of patriarchal society' (Arnold, 1978: 57; see also Hirschon, 1978: 69). The message seems to be that female sexuality is a seething subterranean force which must be brought under stringent discipline if it is not to overwhelm the social order.

This message is not to be found only in feminist theory, however. It lies at the heart of many cultural forms, both 'high' and 'popular', as Kate Millett points out in *Sexual Politics* (Millett, 1977). One example is the popular film *Fatal Attraction* – the titillation and fascination of flirting with female sexual danger lies at the heart of its appeal. In the film wife and mistress represent, respectively, disciplined and uncontrolled female sexuality, and it is significant that Alex (the mistress) uses a carving knife as her weapon – to inflict a symbolic castration using a phallic symbol to which she, as a woman, is not entitled but which, as representative of the archetypal dangerous woman, she usurps. And it is interesting that Alex – note the name – is finally killed not by the 'hero' but by his *wife*; the evil woman's attempt at power is defeated by *female* virtue. In *Fatal Attraction* women provide both protection *and* threat; the *self*-policing of female danger, at first undercut, is in the end sufficient.

So I am not altogether in agreement with Katherine Arnold – women *can*, I would argue, be seen as both willing and able to control themselves. Creating and maintaining feminine self-discipline is the central aim of the ideology of femininity (see e.g. Ferguson, 1983). Self-policing, however, is certainly not sufficient to meet the danger of female sexuality, which is also controlled by law, physical force and through patriarchal ideological constructions of women as weak, dependent and endangered not only by sexual violence but by their own sexuality. The threat remains in spite of all this, however, and this section will analyse the construction of feminine sexuality as ambiguous, focusing on passivity and its shadow, voraciousness, as expressed in the virgin/whore dichotomy. I will argue, following Kate Millett, that the latter element in this construction comes to the fore when feminist struggles directly challenge the social order.

My contention is that underlying both the discourse of feminine sexual disinterest and romantic love lies a discourse – rather than a reality – of a potentially chaotic feminine sexuality, in which penetration is an act fraught with danger. I shall argue that while the behavioural *content* of this virgin/whore dichotomy has changed considerably this century, its *form* remains the same – (self-)discipline threatened by autonomy-as-chaos. On the level of body-concept this dichotomy is expressed in the perception of the inside of the female body simultaneously as empty, open and penetrable space, and as dark, dangerous and engulfing energy.

The feminine object-body, then, has dangerous qualities – it is not wholly passive. This is especially relevant in the current discussion – *how* the object is presented. Eleanor Stephens is among many who have written on female passivity, arguing that women 'have been brought up to play a passive role, and, like Sleeping Beauty, wait patiently for Mr Right to turn the key to our hearts and sexuality' (Stephens, 1976). While this is undoubtedly the case, the construction of women as passive objects is only one side of the story. Looking at strategies of control does not make sense unless we also look at *what they are supposed to control*. We get a hint of this in the presentation of women as the stimulus or precipitator of rape, as an indirect and insidious power/danger. But in representations of sexuality, and especially though not exclusively in pornography (Coward, 1982) we find the most direct articulation of the hidden female bodily power which ideologies of passivity and practices of objectification exist to control.

Penetration as control

Kate Millett argues that the misogynist representations of feminine desire which she identifies in the work of Miller, Mailer and Lawrence formed part of a 'counter-revolution' to the feminism of the late nineteenth and early twentieth centuries (Millett, 1977). Her argument is in many ways similar to Barker-Benfield's analysis of the birth of gynaecological surgery in the late nineteenth century, and has areas of agreement with the feminist analyses of the new reproductive technologies and sexual violence discussed above. What Barker-Benfield and Petchesky argue about medical penetration of the dark interior of woman is essentially what Millett argues about sexual penetration: that masculine penetration of the feminine interior is understood as conquest.

Barker-Benfield and Millett share in common the argument that this penetration responds to a specific feminist threat to the patriarchal social order, and is justified through a definition of women as potentially sexually voracious. Further, both argue that such penetration is understood as an act fraught with danger: a heroic journey into the unknown.

Cora Kaplan questions Millett's historical periodization; she argues that Millett's 'dating of the disappearance of overt misogyny is fuzzy' and asks 'Did it ever disappear?' (Kaplan, 1986: 20). She goes on to suggest that Millett oversimplifies not only in her timing of revolution and counter-revolution but also in her too close identification of 'author, protagonist and point of view' and her lack of acknowledgement of textual ambiguities. All of this allows Millett to suggest that the sexual representations in her chosen texts form a conscious and conspiratorial response to feminism (ibid.: 24, 29). Thus, Kaplan argues, Millett posits mechanical and determinist relationships between politics and ideology, ideology and literature.

I would accept much of Kaplan's critique of Millett. It would be crude and simplistic to argue that their male characters can be read as direct expressions of these writers' politics or behaviour, or that such representations form a conscious anti-feminist conspiracy. Further, it is somewhat problematic to argue that perceptions of feminine sexual danger can slot in and out of history as simple alternatives, since such perceptions are conceptually interdependent with constructions of feminine sexuality as passive. Millett's position on these points *is* ambiguous, and her use of the literary evidence is somewhat mechanical at times. However, she does also argue that the sexual representations under discussion should be seen as 'power fantasy' rather than simple reflections of actual behaviour; she describes them as 'illusory' (Millett, 1977: 21).

I use her analysis, then, in that context; as a discussion of one possible 'resolution' of, rather than *the* patriarchal reaction to the tensions and upheavals feminist struggles cause in a patriarchal society. While it is simplistic to suggest that misogyny 'appears' and 'disappears' from culture I would suggest that we can argue that the usually covert perception of feminine sexuality as dangerous is more directly engaged with ideologically at times when feminism seeks to challenge women's social powerlessness, and that literature is one place where we might look for such engagements. With these caveats in mind, then, I would suggest that Millett's analysis can be used to illuminate the social meanings of feminine sexuality and the feminine body, especially in showing us how the virgin/whore dichotomy resonates on the level of the body.

Before returning to Millett, however, I would like to explore in more depth the argument that the virgin/whore dichotomy, usually associated with specifically Victorian values, is still central in the construction and control of feminine sexuality in contemporary society.

Nice girls do: a sexual revolution?

Lucy Bland argues that since the last century there have been significant changes in the categories through which female sexuality is understood:

> By the late 1960s, with its so-called sexual revolution premarital sex (lesbianism was still taboo) was more possible, more legitimate for young women and girls. As *Vanity Fair* put it in 1971: 'Nice girls do.'
>
> (Bland, 1981: 62)

Bland, like Barker-Benfield, argues that the nineteenth-century ideal of 'asexual' womanhood 'co-existed with other representations, giving a highly contradictory construction of female sexuality' (ibid.: 57–8). She argues that 'the central polarity virgin/whore', through which female sexuality was understood, changed in focus in the nineteenth century, suggesting that the polarity previously seen as innate in all women was then used to *distinguish* the pure, asexual bourgeois wife and 'the impure whore', with the latter being 'the repository of those unacceptable desires and sexual behaviour whose displacement kept the virtuous woman and the home she inhabited pure and unsullied' (ibid.: 59).

While I would substantially accept this analysis, I would argue that it would be more accurate to see the virgin/whore distinction *between* women as an addition to, rather than a replacement of, the idea of the virgin and the whore both battling it out in the one body. Women's greater moral and sexual purity was posited in spite of their greater 'animality', or domination by their reproductive capacities, where women were thought to be continually under the threat of a complete reproductive 'take-over' (ibid.: 58; Ehrenreich and English, 1979: 108). What Barker-Benfield's work shows, I would argue, is that feminine animality could mean not only domination by the womb but also referred, in a more covert fashion, to a feminine sexuality seen as insatiable, which underlay even the bourgeois woman's sexless state.

Bland argues that the sexual revolution must be seen in the context of the Victorian virgin/whore dichotomy. What changed is *content* rather than *form* – to the 'new-style virgin/whore dichotomy . . .[of] the monogamous woman versus the promiscuous' (Bland, 1981: 62). Contemporary ideas about feminine sexuality express the same polarities of discipline/chaos, integrity/openness, subject/object, since female sexuality is still created as heterosexual, dependent and responsive.

Bland argues that monogamy/responsibility is placed as the opposite to promiscuity in 'a reconstructed double standard around promiscuity' (ibid.: 62). The monogamous one-man woman must be sexually responsible – that is, faithful – in controlling fertility and the 'health' risks of non-monogamous sex. Here, Bland argues, the 'cleanliness/filth' polarity central to the distinction of virgin and whore is expressed in medicalized terms (ibid.: 63). Discussing the 'Yorkshire Ripper' she points out that he used the polarity very directly, describing the prostitutes who were his main victims as 'scum' and 'mucky women'; further, she argues that his distinction of innocent and guilty victims was widely unquestioned, showing that: 'the *motive* for killing prostitutes was self-explanatory . . . it was only the killing of "innocent" women which presented a comprehension problem' (ibid.:64; see also Hollway, 1981; Warde-Jouve, 1984; Caputi, 1987).

The virgin/whore dichotomy is still central in the construction of feminine sexuality. Sue Lees has explored its effect on girls' behaviour (Lees, 1986). She argues that the term 'slag' is central in the control of girls' sexuality and behaviour; a 'slag' is a girl who is sexually promiscuous, who sleeps with boys she does not 'love', for active female sexuality 'is rendered safe only when confined to the bonds of marriage and wrapped in the aura of "love"' (ibid.: 28). The only sure protection against this stigmatization is to have, or quickly get, a 'steady' boyfriend (ibid. 36); that is, to validate (possible) sexual activity by becoming exclusive sexual property. Girls cannot themselves initiate sex, but are responsible for boys' sexual behaviour (ibid.: 164). If a girl is known to have slept with 'too many' boys, her property value falls: she becomes 'second-hand' (ibid.: 46), probably sexually voracious (ibid.: 46–8) and definitely indiscriminate, a girl who will 'go with anyone anywhere' (ibid.: 150).

The term 'slag', however, often bears little or no relation to actual sexual behaviour, and is used to constrain girls' actions in non-sexual situations too; its 'vacuousness and ambiguity' allows the term to be used as a general mechanism of control (ibid.: 25, 34, 138–9). Its control, further, operates indirectly, as *self*-control; Lees argues:

> 'Slag' is present as sexual censure even when boys are out of sight and out of mind. Such is the power of male dominance that its exercise is not dependent on the presence of the oppressor . . . I am reminded of the concept of power as 'self-carried', which has been elaborated by Foucault, a power of male dominance which is not 'exercised' by boys over girls, but which girls carry with them and which penetrates their lives and their recreations.
>
> (ibid.: 82)

Although girls must avoid being stigmatized as slags, they must not go too far in the opposite direction and be labelled 'tight', that is, 'unapproachable, sexually cold – a tight bitch' (ibid.: 37). Lees quotes 'Pat': 'It's a vicious circle. If you don't like them, then they'll call you a tight bitch. If you go with them they'll call you a slag afterwards' (ibid.: 37). Lees concludes that in spite of an increase in pre-marital sex, 'the double standard of sexual morality is just as strong today' (ibid.: 167). Bland argues that the distinction goes 'beyond' common sense to institutional use – she cites the centrality of supposed promiscuity and 'moral danger' in understandings and treatment of adolescent girls' 'delinquency' (Bland, 1981: 64; see also Hudson, 1984). And we have seen above how these categorizations operate in the area of sexual violence. As Hirschon points out, then, the social control of women is exerted both externally, through social convention, and internally, as a moral force expressed in the concepts of 'shame' and 'modesty' (Hirschon, 1978: 67).

Women are responsible for sexual control, and can 'precipitate' sexual action through the 'presentation of herself as promiscuous, as sexually available' but they are not themselves independently sexually active (Bland, 1981: 65). Bland concludes:

Thus, in effect, women are not only held responsible for their own sexual behaviour, the consequences of that behaviour, the potential 'health risk', the potential 'dysgenic' breeding . . . they are frequently also held responsible for *male* sexual behaviour.

(ibid.: 64)

Women do not – or ought not – instigate sexually but function as sexual stimulus for masculine action, and are responsible for controlling access to the female body as a stimulating environment. Dominant representations create women as sexual objects for men (ibid.: 65–6). Further, Bland argues that in (many) pornographic representations, 'women's bodies are used as objects of humiliation and loathing', their genitals especially being 'filthy and polluting' (ibid.: 66).

Dangerous bodies

The ensuing discussion of ideas on sexuality in general and pornographic representations in particular seeks to make a number of points. First, I will argue that the central issue of sexuality remains an understanding of man as subject and woman as object. Sexual liberation, as many feminists have pointed out, did not result in sexual autonomy for women, and women's bodies remain an environment on which the masculine subject acts. Further, independent female sexuality and female ownership of the body are engaged with ideologically in pornographic representations (and elsewhere) as the danger and control of female sexual voraciousness and promiscuity. What *has* changed, I would argue, is the *response* to the threat of feminine 'openness'. In place of the nineteenth-century control through denial of the existence of female sexual desire and sexual surgery we can uncover the control of voraciousness through a conceptualization of penetration as possession, exhaustion and repletion. Instead of controlled infusions of sperm, feminine sexuality is contained by exhausting it.

To return, then, to Kate Millett: what does her work tell us about the perception of the feminine body as housing dangerous sexual energies? Millett argues that in 'counter-revolutionary' literature women, and women's bodies, were defined as 'a terrible void, a lack, a deficiency of being within' which only phallic penetration could fill (Millett, 1977: 263, 241). One of the texts Millett discusses is Miller's *Sexus*; she argues that its feminine characters are presented as objects, that Miller:

> converts woman to 'cunt' – thing, commodity, matter. There is no personality to recognize or encounter . . . the perfect woman is a floating metonymy, pure cunt, completely unsullied by human mentality.
>
> (ibid.: 297; 300)

The perfect woman, however, is the *result* of phallic action; before it she has a will, however degraded – she acts. Afterwards she is the perfect will-less, passive object. In *Sexus* the hero, 'Val', recounts his conquest and humiliation of 'Ida', a friend's unfaithful wife. Ida is a vain, deceitful and souless 'monster' who:

> lived entirely in the body, in her senses, her desires – and she directed the show, with her tyrannical little will . . . Ida swallowed everything like a pythonness. She was heartless and insatiable.
>
> (quoted in Millett, 1977: 4)

The rationale of the episode, is, however, to show the *limits* of female insatiability – it can be conquered: in sex with Val, Ida's 'tyrannical little will' entirely disappears and she is totally under his control: 'she was just like a bitch in heat, biting me all over, panting, gasping, wriggling like a worm on the hook' (quoted in ibid.: 3).

Ida aims to control Val and fails; Val aims to humiliate her, to punish her for her 'nymphomania' and destroy her will, and succeeds. Millett argues that 'his penis is now an instrument of chastisement . . . Ida's genitalia are but the means of her humiliation' (ibid.: 7). Her will is destroyed in her reduction to 'paroxysms of sensual capitulation' (ibid.: 8). She is reduced from human to animal status. Since, however, Ida, as a nymphomaniac, 'lived entirely in the body, in her senses, her desires', destroying her will, removing her potential to act independently, merely reduces her to her true status (quoted in ibid.: 4).

As Andrea Dworkin points out in *Intercourse*, the assertion of will, or active and independent desire cannot coexist with the status of sexual object, for 'objects do not will, and want, and search, and are not subjects in a human quest for love or affection or sex' (Dworkin, 1987: 17–18). Ida's independent will is annihilated in sex – she wants only what he wants – her dependent desires make her a helpless object. As Dworkin points out, then, 'the eroticism of the female exists within the bounds of male sexual imperatives' (Dworkin, 1981: 34). Crucially for the present argument, however, this annihilation of feminine subjecthood does not come easy; it depends on an elaboration of sexual acts impossible in reality but realizable in fantasy – the fantasy of a 'potency . . . superb and overwhelming' (Dworkin, 1987: 7–8).

In this fantastic resolution of danger, masculine sexuality is, Millett argues, 'clinical', 'fastidious', a 'self-conscious detachment' (Millett, 1977: 306, 297). She quotes Miller's Val: 'except for the part of me that was in her I was cool as a cucumber and remote as the Dog Star' (quoted in ibid.: 297). He is all self-possession; in contrast, she:

> wasn't any longer a woman in heat, she wasn't even a woman; she was just a mass of indefinable contours wriggling and squirming like a piece of fresh bait.
>
> (quoted in ibid.: 297)

Afterwards:

> She went into a convulsion, delirious with joy and pain. Then her legs slid off my shoulders and fell to the floor with a thud. She lay there like a dead one, completely fucked out.
>
> (quoted in ibid.: 306)

Feminine sexuality is, when exercised autonomously, non-human. Millett picks random quotations from Miller's novels which describe feminine desire as animalistic: 'squealing like a stuck pig'; 'like a crazed animal'; 'like a she-animal' or 'a bright voracious animal' (quoted in ibid.: 306). Her 'autonomy', then, is not real: her sexual energies are not exercised by a fully human subject – they control her rather than her controlling them. Feminine animal voraciousness and masculine sexual self-possession exist in the relationship of nature to culture: the latter defines itself through the subordination of the former.

Phallic penetration takes the sting out of feminine desire; its puny attempts at autonomy destroyed, the feminine body is returned to its true object status. Feminine genitalia is a 'crack', a 'wound', a 'gash', 'a slimy hole' – 'but really only emptiness, nothingness, zero' (ibid.: 307–8). If that emptiness had properties, if it independently desired, its status as passive penetrable object would be in danger. Penetration – in which, paradoxically, the masculine body remains entirely separate and detached – exhausts active feminine desire, showing women that they really want to be what they really are: objects which exist to be used.

The threat of the orifice

In pornography the exploration and resolution at the ideological level of the threat of the sexually active woman, expressed in the concept of female sexuality as voracious, is engaged in even more directly. The focus here is on openings: the mouth/throat, womb, anus and especially vagina. Penetration is the central act of pornography, functioning as action, conquest, humiliation, control and containment. In *Pornography: Men Possessing Women* Andrea Dworkin argues that the narrative of resistance then capitulation which characterizes heterosexual pornography acts to contain a female threat by constructing female desire as ultimately responsive rather than autonomous: what she really wants is what he wants – 'the object is allowed to desire if she desires to be an object' (Dworkin, 1981: 109, 128, 205). This is one way in which the danger of feminine desire is 'resolved' – rendered dependent and responsive. Women do desire, but their desires conveniently and unthreateningly dovetail with 'masculine' desire.

I would argue, however, that this 'resolution' is no longer seen as sufficient. To the issue of what women want sexually is added the question of *how much* they want. In pornographic representations the threat of 'nymphomania' is presented as titillation, flirting with a danger that the endless repetition of pornographic 'plots' has resolved a thousand times before. Dworkin's analysis shows that one penetration is rarely sufficient – variation and repetition forms the sexual crescendo of pornography. It is this feature of pornography which Kate Millett notes – the species of fantasy which Steven Marcus calls 'pornotopic', the 'shower of orgasms' (Millett, 1977: 7). One orgasm is never enough to 'satisfy' – insatiability needs 'a shower of orgasms' to render it safe through exhaustion.

I would argue, then, that constructing feminine desire as the desire of an object to be possessed is only half the resolution which women's 'insatiability' now requires. Also needed are exhaustion and repletion, and the agents of exhaustion are those staple ingredients of pornography, the unnaturally large and inexhaustible penis, and the repetition of sexual acts until both protagonist and audience can be certain that the woman's desires have been exhausted. In 'The Art of Dominating Women' (an illustrated magazine article), for example, we are offered 'intimate details of a thoroughly submissive female and the incredible excesses she requires for total satisfaction' (Dworkin, 1981: 160–1).

An example from Dworkin's work on pornography will clarify the argument. She analyses *Black Fashion Model* by John Wilson. The 'heroine' of the book is Kelly, the richest and most famous black model in America who, although she appears on film 'a wanton, lusty *woman*', is in reality – or so she thinks – innocent (ibid.: 210). The plot, such as it is, hinges on Kelly's abduction and repeated sexual abuse by two men and one woman. The innocent Kelly at first struggles and protests, but she is ultimately unable to resist the pleasure of forced sex: 'Kelly is "beginning to go out of her mind with the powerful affects (sic) of cunt-licking lust!" . . . an inner voice with masochistic urges is telling her that she loves being forced' (ibid.: 212).

Voyeurism and lesbian 'rape' form the hors d'oeuvre; penetration is the entrée:

> Robert Gray fingerfucks her. He keeps withdrawing. He spreads the fluid from her cunt on his cock with his fingers. He tells her it excites her. His monstrous white shaft is between her black thighs. His fingers pinch her clitoris. He puts his finger in her. Robert Gray's 'blood-filled cock would soon be ramming into her body' . . . when his cock is buried in her belly she feels as though she is being stretched apart. She loves it . . . She is hopelessly impaled.
>
> (ibid.: 213)

The excitement comes from her continual attempts to resist – at first to resist the acts, then to resist enjoying them. Of course, both prove impossible: her 'hot little gash seemed to gape in greedy desire'. Robert Gray, by contrast, remains completely in control – he can stop and start at will and keep going for as long as he chooses, indeed, until Kelly 'finally goes limp . . . her body was beaten and bruised and satiated from the ravishment' (ibid.: 214).

Not quite satiated enough, however, it turns out. The final course is a black man with a penis 'too big for any natural orifice' (ibid.: 214). Robert Gray – now not quite 'monstrous' enough, it would seem – having dealt with her vagina, 'Bart Kurtis' takes over:

> He makes her suck . . . His cock keeps sticking at the bottom of her throat. She feels lust . . . Bart lunges viciously in her throat but she is sucking with wild abandon. Her pain is horrible but her lust is overwhelming.
>
> (ibid.: 214)

Anal rape finishes Kelly's humiliation: 'it is like a crucifixion, "the nail pounding into her . . . defiling her asshole". Then she starts to get excited and like it . . . Kelly cums and cums and cums' (ibid.: 215).

In her discussion of *Whip Chick*, a story of female sadism, Dworkin argues that 'in fantasy, the male can experiment with the consequences as he imagines them of loss of power over women' (ibid.: 35). I would argue that experimentation with fear and danger does not rely on the explicit presentation of feminine sexuality as openly sadistic. What the discussion of *Black Fashion Model* shows is that even the superficially innocent one-man woman presents a threat; all feminine desire is dangerous and must be made dependent, its active, willed elements removed and its potential exhausted. As Dworkin points out, *Black Fashion Model* is a profoundly racist text; its 'heroine', as a black woman in a white milieu, is doubly powerless as well as doubly sexualized. In spite of this, her 'desire' is dangerous, and must be exhausted.

Independent female desire, even when not openly sadistic and castrating, still threatens the gender order of subject and object, actor and environment, by its very existence. On the level of the body, insatiability and the threat of disorder rest in bodily orifices – hot, gaping and greedy 'gashes'. Represented as fundamentally open and penetrable, openness is the bodily locus of weakness, vulnerability and incompletion, the passive orifices through which women are conquered and possessed by the active male; as 'The Art of Dominating Women' tells us, 'fucked by a big dick until there was hardly a hole left' (ibid.: 163). However, the deeper meaning of openness and incompletion, seldom articulated, emerges into view as what makes conquest to the point of exhaustion necessary. Feminine incompletion is ambiguously constructed so that masculine desire, represented by the penis, is all that is needed to complete it – but this completion is far from secure. The pornographic fantasy of the inhumanly large and inexhaustible penis, I would argue, shows us the insecurity of masculine conquest and ownership as well as the definition of feminine bodily openness as weakness. The other side of penetration is, as Dworkin describes, the fear of being engulfed in 'the burying, enveloping, suffocating, killing quality of sex with a woman' (Dworkin, 1987: 24), in 'the voracious cunts of pornography' (Dworkin, 1981: 224).

The feminine body: objectification, discipline and chaos

The definitions of active/masculine and passive/feminine operate in a dependent opposition; if one changes, both change. As Dworkin argues, 'the first rule of masculinity is that whatever he is, women are not' (Dworkin, 1981: 50). Feminine desire must be contained by responsiveness, and the danger of independent, active and autonomous feminine desire is controlled in reality by stringent sanctions and social disgust; and resolved in fantasy by annihilation of the will and exhaustion of desire. Women's empty inner space must be policed in reality and filled up in fantasy. Women's bodily appetites, if not controlled, threaten chaos. As Dworkin argues, 'in the male sexual framework the sadistic whore whose sexuality is murderous and insatiable ultimately . . . is also the exquisite victim, fulfilled through annihilation' (ibid.: 176). She is fulfilled; she wants no more; she wants only what he chooses to give. Penetration equals conquest and possession, but a conquest and possession so insecure that they must be forever repeated.

Feminine desire responds to something outside of itself, while masculine desire comes from within and satisfies itself through the responsive feminine environment. The masculine body is complete in itself. The feminine body is empty until filled by men. Emptiness, however, represents both weakness and danger.

Women, however, strive to be both female *and* human. Thus, they must act, but still respond. They must be independent but still dependent, active, but not too active, passive, but not too passive, self-contained but still open. The ultimate irreconcilability of acting like a woman while thinking oneself an individual is expressed on the level of the body in the struggle to impose an impenetrable cosmetic facade and an autonomous sexuality – a sexual boundary – on a body whose definition centres on orifices: the open mouth of advertising, the voracious vagina of pornography, the Freudian genitalia as wound, the inner space of Erikson's psychology.

The struggle is to contain the desire and the chaos which those orifices symbolize, to remain on the right side of the virgin/whore divide, to show that self-control is possible. Women must safeguard their bodies, their emotions and their sexuality as masculine property, as caretakers of objects produced for masculine consumption. They must maintain a physical integrity which the definition of their bodies as open continually undercuts. The smooth surface must look impenetrable but can never really be impenetrable. The impossibility of ever really becoming 'persons' must stay hidden in the continual struggle to be both person and woman.

As we saw in Chapters 2 and 3, reconciling individuality and independence with femininity and responsiveness in the 'correct' way is presented by psychiatry and, to a lesser extent, by feminist therapists, as the ultimate cure for anorexia. The next chapter argues that articulating the demands of individuality and femininity is precisely what the anorexic woman aims to do through her control of eating and appetite which she describes in exactly the terms used to describe feminine sexuality – as animalistic and potentially overwhelming. She does this during, rather than after, the illness. In this chapter I have tried to show how the definition of the female body in bourgeois culture operates through the concepts of object, discipline and chaos; in the final chapters the articulation of these concepts in anorexia will be analysed.

Chapter 7

The anorexic symptom

Nicky Diamond argues that our ideas about the body 'are not simply references to properties of anatomy, but produce a social phantom body-anatomy which is structured in form and inscribed with magical, imaginary properties' (Diamond, 1985: 57). Some 'imaginary properties' of the feminine body were analysed in the previous chapter which attempted to outline the dominant social meanings which construct that body in bourgeois patriarchal culture. Here the three central axes of meaning were explored.

First, the feminine body is created as an object on which the masculine subject acts, and which he owns; women maintain their bodies as objects through dietary, cosmetic and behavioural practices as caretakers rather than owners. Thus, I would argue, Turner's assertion that women have a 'phenomenological possession' of their bodies sits uneasily with women's alienation from their bodies as the objects of masculine sexual desire and the site of personally uncontrolled reproduction. Second, self-control is, as we have seen, an essential feature of femininity and of women's relationship with their bodies: women watch what they eat, how they dress, talk, sit, walk and behave. Finally, there is the other side of the coin of self-control – fear and disgust at the appetites which necessitate that control: women's potential to overwhelm the boundaries of femininity and restricted feminine space.

Diamond goes on to argue that the ideas about the body 'in social circulation' are actively engaged with, rather than passively accepted: 'worked with – reproduced and *reworked* by each specific site of image production' (ibid.: 54). In this chapter anorexia will be analysed as a 'site of image production'. I will analyse the reproductions and reworkings of the concepts of the body which take place in anorexia through the concepts of objectification, discipline and chaos.

In anorexia feminine self-control takes on new dimensions. 'Weight-watching' becomes the major, and eventually the sole activity of the anorexic woman. This chapter will examine the ritualized eating pattern through which anorexic self-control is effected, primarily through analysis of the responses to a question-naire completed by 35 anorexic women. What will be argued here is that anorexic rituals attempt to create secure defences against appetite, and that the ultimate goal is the construction of the body as desireless and inviolate. Eating nothing – allowing nothing into the body – is, therefore, the end towards which anorexic rituals aim.

The enemy of anorexic control is appetite. Appetite is the chaos which makes discipline so necessary; appetite is the danger from which ritualized eating tries to protect the self; and appetite is the force which undermines and makes so precarious anorexic self-control. Through an analysis of anorexic women's descriptions of eating I will argue that the concept of feminine insatiability is translated, in anorexia, from sex to food, and the characterization of feminine desire as non-human intensified. Further, the danger that feminine desire will encroach into masculine space, its con-struction as antithetical to patriarchal order, is expressed internally in the anorexic body as appetite (feminine) threatening self (masculine) – a transformation of a public and social inter-gender conflict into a private and individualized intra-gender struggle.

Here the central argument will be that in anorexia the body and its appetites are transformed in an attempt to eradicate desire. This splitting process is, as we shall see, defined by anorexic women in a variety of ways – either the body, food, or the anorexia itself come to be seen as alien. Further, the distinction is one of oppression and control; the conscious strategy of not eating comes to control and oppress its creator. The sense of control by an external force is mirrored in hospitalization, where the anorexic woman becomes the object of medical control. Women's bodily alienation and objectification, then, are transformed in anorexia with the con-struction of an absolute opposition between appetite and 'self'. Here the body is split into two: the desiring body, in which appetite is lodged; and the desireless body, which needs nothing and wants nothing.

In anorexia, then, the social construction of the feminine body through objectification and the discipline/chaos dichotomy is taken to its logical conclusion. Socially these meanings are primarily expressed as sexual, with a secondary expression in dietary self-control versus 'naughty' indulgence as especially meaningful for women. In anorexia, control and insatiability centre primarily around food and eating, with a secondary expression in sexuality. This reversal, I would suggest, can best be explained as *accessibility* – in the privatized reworking of the dominant social meanings of the body which anorexia effects, eating is controllable. The sexual body, as an object, is not.

Anorexia, however, does not simply express and transform social meanings – it also attempts to resolve their contradictions. The anorexic women aims, through a ritualized eating pattern, to create the surface of the feminine body as an *absolute* barrier and the body itself an an *absolute* object. In anorexia the concept of receptivity/penetrability as weakness and incompletion is overcome by creating the body as a self-contained object which takes in nothing from the external environment. Food, here, represents external intrusion: the aim is to eliminate it completely and create a pure, empty and static inner space free from contamination by intrusion.

The anorexic 'shell', then, functions in two senses: to prevent intrusion and to contain emptiness. The barrier of ritual completes feminine incompletion by allowing nothing in, and signifies bodily integrity in the end of penetrability. Feminine bodily openness, however, is more complex in meaning than simple weakness, as we have seen. Penetrability represents incompletion as well as voraciousness and potential encompassment, and *both* meanings are reworked in anorexia in the split between the body as desiring enemy and desireless ally. Hunger in anorexia is symbolic of all desire, and the insatiability of feminine desire is expressed in anorexia by the construction of appetite as a force which must be eliminated if it is not to destroy the 'self'. The barrier-body in anorexia aims, then, at desirelessness and needlessness. Not just food, but the desire for food is dangerous and threatening – the object-body is created to eliminate both. The desiring body, however, continually threatens the elimination of appetite by its desire to take in, to encompass.

The ultimate aim of anorexia is the destruction of the desiring body in which dangerous appetite is lodged, and the ascendancy of the object-body. The aim is to create the body as an absolute object – inviolate, complete, inactive and initiativeless – wholly owned and controlled by the self. The irony of anorexia is that the object-body comes to control the self. As we shall see, in 'second stage' anorexia starvation as a conscious strategy is itself transformed into an oppressor – the anorexic woman feels powerless to stop a process she herself began.

Before going on to look in detail at the questionnaire responses, however, it will be helpful to consider the theoretical issues they raise. I will begin with a discussion of Turner's analysis of anorexia, since my arguments on the social construction of the body are indebted to his work.

TURNER'S SOCIOLOGY OF THE BODY

In Turner's sociology of the body, he argues that each society has four 'tasks' in relation to the body: the reproduction of populations through time; the regulation of bodies in space; the restraint of desire through disciplines; and the representation of the body in social space (Turner, 1984: 2–3, 91). Here illnesses, he argues, especially those of subordinate groups, are 'cultural indications of the problem of control' (ibid.: 2–3). He argues thus:

> since the government of the body is in fact the government of sexuality, the problem of regulation is in practice the regulation of female sexuality by a system of patriarchal power.
>
> (ibid.: 91)

> the control of bodies is essentially the control of female bodies.
>
> (ibid.: 249)

For Turner, certain characteristic illnesses are associated with the four dimensions of the social control of bodies. Women's illnesses especially are diseases of dependency: 'the medical problems of subordinates are products of the political and ideological regulation of sexuality' (ibid.: 92). And this dependency is reinforced and legitimated in treatment. In this system, then, anorexia, as well as being a disorder of dependency is a disease of presentation, associated with the fourth dimension of the regulation of bodies (ibid.: 95). He argues that in modern societies the representation of the body/self is a particularly acute issue, since it is no longer lodged in fixed social roles but is symbolically highly flexible (ibid.:

92; see also 174); anorexia, then, is 'an anxiety directed at the surface of the body in a system organized around narcissistic consumption' (ibid.: 93).

As middle-class women entered public society in the twentieth century female illnesses became increasingly presentational, and 'symbolic of anxieties about the surface of the body' (ibid.: 108). Anorexia 'most dramatically expresses the ambiguities of female gender in contemporary Western societies', in that it expresses both the 'representational crisis' of the individual in late capitalism through the modern view of beauty as thinness and the struggle of women against dependency, the anorexic woman suffering from 'protective parenting in the confines of the privatized family' (ibid.: 113).

Anorexia and bulimia are, then, 'two individualized forms of protest which employ the body as a medium of protest against the consumer-self' (ibid.: 180). Turner suggests that anorexia is a struggle within the middle-class family 'where over-protected [girls] seek greater control over their bodies and therefore their lives', an ascetic control through subordination of the flesh which paradoxically results in the dominance of the body when eating, dieting, food and getting rid of food become 'all-consuming passions' (ibid.: 184). Further, anorexia entails a 'contradictory' sexual symbolism. The anorexic woman rejects sexuality by her suppression of menstruation but at the same time conforms to cultural norms of female attractiveness in her pursuit of thinness (ibid.: 185).

Refusal to eat is, then, for Turner 'an oppostion to parental feeding which gives the child some control over bodily functions' (ibid.: 191). He argues that the 'anorexic' family is characterized by the contradictory demands it places on its daughters. While competitive success, usually educational, is emphasized, compliance, rather than the independence through which success might be gained, is promoted. The 'overpowering, dominant mother' brings up her children to fulfil her interests rather than their own, and thus inadequately prepares the child for adolescensce by stifling individualization (ibid.: 192).

The anorexic daughter chooses her illness as a defence against this confusion. On the one hand, she 'gives in' to compliance by suppressing sexuality and maturity through her suppression of menstruation and adoption of 'a permanently childlike body and attitude to the mother'. On the other, she gains a sense of independent control through her control of food and her body – 'this is her peculiar compelling path to selfhood' (ibid.: 193). It is, then, the mother's control, effected through nurturing, which the anorexic woman seeks to escape – since the anorexic family has a dominant mother and a father who is either weak or absent, it 'suffers from matriarchal not patriarchal control' (ibid.: 196; 195).

However, once she has chosen anorexia, biological processes take over: 'it becomes increasingly difficult to control, interrupt or redirect the process of weight loss, absence of appetite, overactivity, insomnia and amenorrhoea' (ibid.: 193). As well as this, the logic of denial leads to a 'moral spiral': 'the anorexic pattern of asceticism requires obligations which cannot be met so that lapses into self-indulgence are regarded as imperfections which drive her into further reinforcements of the regimen' (ibid.: 194). The anorexic woman chooses her symptom, but then the body takes over: her choice for autonomy results in 'the dominance of nature over culture' (ibid.: 202).

Anorexia is not, however, *wholly* explicable in the familial context for Turner. He argues that a feminist perspective which points to the control of women's bodies through the ideals of beauty and thinness and their commoditization is valuable in that it locates anorexia historically and socially as an illness which, like hysteria in the nineteenth century and depression in the twentieth, expresses 'the structural limitations' placed on women who are at the same time, especially in the middle class, expected to be both feminine and 'successful in the public domain' (ibid.: 196). Anorexia, then, results both from matriarchy in the family and patriarchy in the wider society (ibid.: 197–8; see also 200, 203). There is 'a contradiction between the achievement orientation within the home and the public restraints on female success outside' (ibid.: 201).

CRITIQUE OF TURNER

This is an interesting if somewhat confused analysis of anorexia. First, it works from a number of questionable assumptions about the illness itself. Turner appears to assume that amenorrhoea is one of the main conscious aims of anorexia, and that it expresses a suppression of sexual maturity. I would question whether this is the case. Not only is it unlikely, as Wellbourne and Purgold point out, that the 'pre-anorexic' girl knows enough about biology to realize that starvation will stop menstruation before she embarks on the anorexic process, but also absence of periods can lead to the 'discovery' of anorexia when the anorexic woman becomes concerned about her lack of periods and goes to the doctor (Wellbourne and Purgold, 1984: 35–6). Further, Turner posits a rather simplistic and biologistic link between menstruation and sexuality; menstruation is only *one* of the signs, both social and biological, that an adolescent girl must adjust herself to adult feminine sexuality.

Turner also accepts rather unquestioningly for a sociologist the psychiatric explanation of anorexia as a 'biological take-over', in which the body rather than the woman maintains the illness. It is unfortunate that his more promising idea of a 'moral spiral' is not expanded to counter this. He argues quite wrongly that anorexia entails loss of appetite, and thus suggests that staying anorexic is an easy process. The literature, and, as we shall see, my own material, contradicts both these assumptions. He thus needs only to explain why the anorexic girl begins, not why she keeps going. This is one reason why his explanation of anorexia as a disease of presentation is advanced, since her anxiety about self-presentation and the cultural valuation of feminine thinness provide ample explanation of why so many women diet. We seem almost to be back again with anorexia as 'dieting gone too far'.

Rather more serious, however, is his almost wholesale acceptance of the Bruch theory of pathological families, which was criticized above. Again we find the implication that in a 'proper' family – presumably one with a dominant father and a weak mother? – the conflicts which produce anorexia would be avoidable and 'independence', educational and career success achievable. Although Turner argues that family structures are 'determined' by social structure, and mentions in passing that the 'dominant mother' is herself a product of patriarchy, this social perspective is added on to the Bruch thesis rather than used to criticize it.

If we accept the ideological contradictions between independence as individuals and dependence as women which produce anorexia as a central feature of women's *social* experience in a patriarchal and capitalist society we would expect to find expressions of that contradiction both in the family and in the wider society. As Boskind-Lodahl points out:

the feeling of not having any identity is not a delusion or a misperception but a reality which need not be caused solely by the stereotyped protective mother but by other cultural, social and psychological pressures as well.

(Boskind-Lodahl, 1976: 347)

There are, then, alternatives to attributing 'achievement orientation' to the 'pathological' family with its domineering mother and 'public restraints' – does this mean femininity? – to 'outside' society.

What worries me most, however, is Turner's downgrading of the issue of desire in anorexia by defining it as a disease of presentation. Of course, this analysis allows anorexia to fit very neatly into Turner's four-point plan; I would argue, however, that if the plan did not force us into an either/or choice between the regulation of desire and the representation of the body we might usefully analyse anorexia as expressing both. Turner himself argues that anorexic women 'suppress' sexuality but argues also, rather contradictorily, that an individualized rejection of sexuality conforms to the ideology of sexual expression through personal choice. Quite how anorexia can be seen to make the body 'a vehicle of desire' is not clear. But because Turner thinks that anorexic women are not hungry he ignores the continual struggle with the desire for food which is central in anorexia. Further, he sidesteps the whole issue of what sexual 'choice' can really mean for women in a patriarchal culture.

Turner has followed Foucault throughout his analysis of the body, but he seems to miss out on the potential of this perspective for analysing the differences between masculine and feminine experiences of desire in bourgeois culture. Foucault argues that it is simplistic to see structures of power as suppressing a natural and inherent sexuality; rather, sexualities are produced *through* power/knowledge (Foucault, 1979; 1980). We could use this perspective to argue that masculine desire is produced as active, feminine desire as responsive. Thus, for men being fit for pleasure is being fit to act; for women it is being fit to be *acted on*. Further, such a perspective could be used to prevent us treating masculine sexuality as the unanalysed norm from which feminine sexuality deviates. If we see desire as a socially created force rather than a socially repressed natural appetite then we can see that masculine as well as feminine sexuality, male as well as female bodies are regulated and controlled in culture.

Presentation is vital and anxiety-producing specifically for women, as women must produce desirable bodies, but so also is the self-control of feminine sexuality as responsive rather than active. Here the conflict between individuality and femininity is again central: the formal gender-neutrality of the ideology of individualism suggests that women, as well as men, can be independent, active and pleasure-seeking. However, this is undercut for women by the ideology of femininity which creates women as dependent, passive and the sought rather than the seeker. Desire, therefore, is fundamentally problematical for women, who must reconcile as persons and as bodies these contradictions. Anorexia, I would argue, is one such attempt to reconcile the irreconcilable at the level of the body, and is thus explicitly a disease of desire as well as a disease of presentation.

I would argue, then, that we can use Turner's general perspective on the sociology of the body without necessarily reaching quite the same conclusions, on anorexia at least. And it is to such an analysis that we now turn.

DISCIPLINE

As we have seen, the need to achieve a sense of mastery, or control, has been seen as central in the development of anorexia by, especially, Hilde Bruch and Marilyn Lawrence. Bruch locates the need for control in faulty upbringing, Lawrence in a social structure which denies women autonomy in many areas of their lives. My acceptance of the latter view was explained above, and will figure in further discussion, but for the present, I would like to look at how anorexic women see the issue of control, the ritualized eating pattern through which the attempt to maintain control is organized, and the threat of chaos against which the attempt struggles, and which explains, for anorexic women, its necessity.

In the questionnaire, I asked the women to explain, if they could, why they think they became anorexic. Their explanations were offered tentatively in the main, against a background of uncertainty not infrequently amounting to bafflement. However, the need to exert some control over something in an environment in which the woman feels powerless was a dominant explanatory strand.[1]

The conscious aim of the control of food and weight is achievement; through the control mastery, power and success will, it is expected, be gained, and will be evident to the world around her and especially to the people she feels are trying to dominate her. The question, then, was 'Why do you think you became anorexic?':

> Throughout my childhood, I had done exactly what was asked of me, and was held up to be the 'perfect' child. At about 17, there was conflict about my future [school, college, career etc.] and I gave in to parents' wishes, but started my own social life, with my first sexual encounters, and at this time, the dieting also began.
>
> (Sophie)

> I felt my younger sister was the apple of my (warring) parents' eye and that I was a failure. I had to take a stand and control *something*.
>
> (Sheila)

> a streak of perfectionism . . . probably family expectations, fear of growing up, academic pressures, and the need to do *something* well all played a part . . . Often I still feel I somehow *have* to be slimmer than all my friends. This is irrational I know.
>
> (Irene)

> an excessive case of self-discipline . . . a need to control something when my whole future [career, relationships, etc.] broke down and a move away from home which coincided with all this.
>
> (Andrea)

> I felt unsafe and insecure in a big and threatening world . . . the anorexia was a way of coping and an escape from a world that I felt I couldn't cope with.
>
> (Jane)

> I . . . felt that only being super-slim and attractive would warrant my success as a person.
>
> (Barbara)

The cause of the sense of powerlessness, which leads to control, is explained most often as parental control and expectations, but also as pressure from friends, the school, the anorexic woman's own high expectations of herself and 'the world' itself.

Feminists (and others) have argued that the family is the primary location of the social control of women, the social institution in which patriarchal constraints are transmitted and are most directly felt. An acceptance of this argument, however, should not lead us to argue that the family is the *only* source of patriarchal control and the 'cause' of the oppression of women. Rather, the family is one institution through which patriarchal social control operates; the expectations and world-views of friends, school and the culture in general, the sexual division of labour and the institution of heterosexuality all produce and reproduce the ideology of femininity. It is perhaps understandable, though, that in an individualist culture explanations of powerlessness should be sought in personal and familial relationships rather than in a social structure which produces women as relatively powerless, economically, psychologically, socially, sexually and politically.

Once a need for control has been identified, then, how is that need acted on? For the respondents diet is the *obvious* arena of control for women; the questionnaire responses simply take it for granted, and not surprisingly also take thinness as a feminine ideal:

> The only independence I could have was to be independent of food and no-one could make me change.
>
> (Anne)

> I became anorexic as a result of dieting which I couldn't stop. However much weight I lost I just wanted to lose more. I am 5 ft 6½ ins tall, and my goal weight was 6 stone (I never achieved this weight). I felt more attractive the slimmer I became, and felt more confident and controlled. I felt I was displaying supreme self-control. The slimmer I became the more successful in everything I felt.
>
> (Paula)

> I needed to have something in my life which I was in control of . . . I felt that by limiting my food intake I was gaining a sense of power.
>
> (Frances)

> I feared failure and felt my life was out of control. All I could control was my weight. I *think* those are the reasons but therapy might lead me to new possibilities.
>
> (Patricia)

As we saw in the previous chapter, dieting is a major element in feminine self-control and, as well as expressing the value of restraint for women, in dieting the body is also worked on as a major element in the construction of a 'cosmetic exterior'. The concern with eating and the body shows what areas of their lives women *can* control. Women's involvement with food shows the extent and the nature of the responsibilities of the female role. Ardener describes this as women's 'petty time-consuming activity' (Ardener, 1978: 16); part of the powerlessness of women is their ghettoization in activities seen as trivial.

In the previous chapter we looked at the importance of 'beauty' in femininity, and the role which dieting plays there. But food is more generally women's business. As Rhian Ellis argues, 'from an early age girls are taught to cook for and how to serve food to men' (Ellis, 1983: 165). And as Murcott points out, cooking is women's responsibility: 'cooking is securely anchored as the responsibility of women as wives and mothers . . . the kitchen was their domain' (Murcott, 1983b: 181). It's not, Murcott points out, that men never cook; as Oakley found out in her studies of housework (Oakley, 1974), men 'help' with what is primarily a female responsibility. However, 'it is always women who daily, routinely, and as a matter of course are to do the cooking' (Murcott, 1983c: 82).

The convention of who cooks for whom expresses, Ellis argues, 'wider issues of male authority'; women cooking for men expresses men's power over women's time and labour, and Ellis quotes a remark from the Dobash (1980) study of marital violence to illuminate her point: 'She'll have my tea ready when I go into this house, not when she feels like it' (Ellis, 1983: 166, 169). Food is women's responsibility, then, but women's responsibility as subordinates. Murcott found in her research that women cook mainly according to their husband's preferences rather than their own, and argues that 'their responsibility in this sphere is tempered with references to their husband's, not their own, choice . . . in a literal expression of wives' deference to husband's authority' (Murcott, 1983c: 79–80, 89). Although buying, preparing, cooking and serving food is women's work, women do not control their labour; Murcott argues that while women are responsible for doing the work of cooking, 'they are answerable to the person in whom the power to delegate is originally vested' (ibid.: 89).

Food, then, is one of the ways in which, in Gamarnikow and Purvis's phrase, men are 'the recipients and controllers of female servicing' (Gamarnikow and Purvis, 1985: 3; see also Imray and Middleton, 1983: 23). For women, cooking is primarily a service for others, principally men and children. Murcott found that her respondents felt that cooking for oneself was not worth the time and effort, and that when women are alone they: '"pick" at something that happens to be in the house, have a bar of chocolate or packet of crisps later in the evening or a snack' (Murcott, 1983c: 84). A 'proper' dinner – a cooked meal of meat, potatoes, vegetables and gravy – is for other people; the labour it necessitates is not worth it for women alone. Murcott concludes that 'if husbands and children are absent, women alone will not "cook", indeed many may not even eat' (ibid.: 85, 80–4). Food for women, then, expresses the priority of others' needs and wants rather than personal desire. Cooking is for others, the dictates of personal tastes unimportant, and dieting normal.

With this in mind, the 'choice' of anorexic women to seek control through eating is perhaps as obvious to the reader as it is to them. Once diet has been 'chosen' as the way to achieve mastery and success, a complex set of rituals around food and eating specifically, and the body and its environment generally, is developed.

Mary Douglas defines ritual as 'an attempt to create and maintain a particular culture, a particular set of assumptions by which experience is controlled' (Douglas, 1966: 128). Ritual frames experience; 'the marked-off time or place alerts a special kind of expectancy . . . framing and boxing limit experience, shut in desired themes or shut out intruding ones' (ibid.: 63).

She argues that the ritual behaviour of 'primitive' societies should be differentiated from modern ritual acts not on grounds of sophistication or 'real' knowledge of scientific truth, but because primitive cultures are unified cultures, and modern cultures are fragmented (ibid.: 2, 35, 68–9). In primitive cultures 'the same set of ever more powerful symbols' is used in every context; what is included and excluded, what is seen as dangerous or polluting is the same for the whole society. In modern societies, experience is fragmented, rituals express different inclusions and exclusions and create 'a lot of little sub-worlds, unrelated' (ibid.: 69).

Modern justification for purification, or dirt avoidance rituals as necessitated by 'hygiene' is often, Douglas argues, based on 'fantasy' (ibid.: 69); the fundamentals of modern cleanliness rituals were established *before* bacteriology. Douglas argues thus:

> if we . . . abstract pathogenicity and hygiene from our notions
> of dirt, we are left with the old definition of dirt as matter out
> of place . . . where there is dirt there is system. Dirt is the
> by-product of a systematic ordering and classification of matter,
> in so far as ordering involves rejecting inappropriate elements.
> This idea of dirt takes us straight into the field of symbolism.
>
> (ibid.: 35)

Dirt, then, represents disorder, matter out of place; its elimination
is thus 'a positive effort to organise the environment' in order to
conform to the dominant categorizations of experience; 'our pollution behaviour is the reaction which condemns any object or idea
likely to confuse or contradict cherished classifications' (ibid.: 36).
Ritual 'arises from the interplay of form and surrounding formlessness. Pollution dangers strike when form has been attacked'
(ibid.: 104).

This understanding of ritual can fruitfully be used in the
analysis of anorexia. Three features of Douglas's thesis are especially relevant: ritual, she suggests, frames and controls experience
through the inclusion of what is safe and valued and the exclusion
of what is dangerous or polluting; it does this by defining as
polluting/dangerous that which crosses the lines between order
and formlessness; and in modern societies rituals express the
fragmented experience of discrete social groups. In anorexia, the
ritual practices with which women surround the act of eating
function to allow into the body/system 'safe' food and exclude
'dangerous' food. The restricted list of allowed food, the control
of time, place and manner of eating impose order on a threatened
chaos of appetite which is most directly present in the act of eating.

Douglas argues that 'transitional states' are dangerous because
transition is 'neither one state nor the next, it is indefinable' (ibid.:
96). Eating in anorexia is precisely such a transitional state –
between emptiness and purity and fullness and shame, between
the denial of appetite and surrendering to it. The order which
anorexic rituals impose on each act of eating attempts to control
the formlessness of appetite. Now, while it would be wholly inac-
curate to define 'normal' or non-anorexic eating as 'unritualized',
it *is*, however, clear that anorexic eating is much more densely and
consciously ritualized than the three meal a day status quo. While
'non-anorexic' eating is certainly not determined by response to a
'natural' appetite – we do not eat only when we are hungry and

exactly what we want – it does allow for some 'responsive' eating – snacks or eating between meals. Non-anorexic eating is disciplined, for example, by the structure of the working day, but it also allows some flexibility. For the non-anorexic the world won't come to an end through eating between meals, or eating something new or unusual. For the anorexic woman *all* eating is dangerous and transitional, and ritualization is an attempt to make it progressively safer by divesting it as far as possible of spontaneity and response to desire. It is, in fact, *appetite*, the desire for food which is dangerous, which represents formlessness; the anorexic woman fears that once she starts to eat she will be unable to stop in a chaos of appetite. The daily plan of eating the same food in the same place at the same time in the same way reduces the possibility that appetite will break into her order.

If it were as simple as all food being wholly negative, however, the anorexic dilemma would be simple and fatal. Appetite, however, is both dangerous *and* pleasurable. At the start of the anorexic process only certain foods are defined as polluting – usually 'fattening' or 'forbidden' foods. Foods defined in the dominant discourses of nutrition and diet as allowable and virtuous are 'safe' – that is, non-polluting. The distinction here is between food as *fuel* and food as *pleasure*. Thus far, anorexic categorizations follow dominant social ideas about food, albeit far more rigidly. But the category of 'safe' food is hard to maintain.

The anorexic woman is continually hungry, and the danger of that hunger is too great to be wholly contained by the exclusion of the obviously forbidden. Douglas argues that 'the quest for purity' pursued through a rejection of disorder is paradoxical; experience is not amenable to 'logical categories of non-contradiction', it does not 'tidily fit into accepted categories'. She argues that total purity in experiential categories is impossible, and that we must either accept this, or blind ourselves to the inadequacy of our concepts to totally contain experience (ibid.: 162, 163).

For the anorexic woman, purity in food categories is never wholly possible, for it is not the inherent properties of the food itself which are dangerous, but her desire for it. She can reduce the danger of that desire by eliminating the foods she desires most, but she can never totally eliminate the desire entailed in hunger. As she eats from a more and more restricted list of foods, appetite attaches itself to originally *less* dangerous foods which themselves must then be eliminated. The aim is to reduce the danger by

cutting out more and more foods; the 'dangerous' category, therefore, continually expands while the safe category contracts. The
ultimate aim of anorexia is to eat nothing at all, and the fact that
few women ever attain this does not make it less of an ideal. For
most the rituals are far from perfect; they *lessen* the danger of
appetite rather than abolish it. Most anorexic women are forced
to accept that not eating at all is not a real possibility: the aim of
anorexia is not death, but living with a complete physical integrity
maintained through the absence of desire.

To that degree, then, in spite of what is said about their
'inability' to perceive complexities and 'grey' areas (see Chapter 2
above), anorexic women do tolerate ambiguity. But this tolerance
is never comfortable, because it is not secure. No matter how little
they eat, or how virtuous and pleasure-free their allowed foods,
hunger still remains and perpetually threatens their control.

The central difference between anorexic ritual and ritual as
Douglas defines it is that the latter is social in both meaning and
practice, while the former is social in meaning but individualized
in practice.

The previous chapter suggested that when patriarchal power is
threatened, female desire is defined as dangerous and/or polluting. Indeed, Douglas notes this, arguing that when patriarchy is
secure, it is maintained by sanctions rather than pollution rules.
When dominance is threatened, the sense of its precariousness is
expressed through definitions of danger and pollution. She argues
that this 'Delilah complex' – the idea that women and female
sexuality weaken and betray men/society – occurs in cultures
where women *do* have the power to weaken men, in the culture 'at
war with itself' (ibid.: 140–54). I have suggested in the previous
chapter that the 'Delilah complex' is currently a dominant strand
in sexual politics.

For the anorexic woman dangerous sexuality and its potential
to overwhelm is transformed into desire for food, an arena in
which control and containment is, as we have pointed out, both
accessible and possible. But while belief in the potential danger of
feminine desire is socially created and maintained in ideology the
anorexic woman maintains her transformed definition of danger
alone. Collective danger is not counteracted by collective ritual in
anorexia; rather, collective danger is counteracted by individual
practice. This, I would argue, is why Douglas' argument that
formlessness is seen both as dangerous and potentially creative of

new order (ibid.: 94–5) is not applicable in anorexic ritual, where the danger of formlessness and the protective order of ritual occur in the one body.

In anorexia the threat of formlessness, or a chaos of appetite, is not a threat on the self from 'outside', but operates within the self, where its social power appears as individual. It is the anorexic woman's integrity which desire will destroy, since that integrity rests on desirelessness. Operating *against* social definitions of the feminine body as incomplete, this construction is forever precarious. The struggle between feminine desire and patriarchal order, carried on internally, represents only danger, devoid of creative potential.

The anorexic system is a system at war with itself. The struggle takes place inside one body which represents both danger and order. In social ritual, the fear of dangerous impurities entering the social system express a fear of danger from without (ibid.: 121–2); in anorexic ritual the impurity, as appetite, is internal and can only partially be externalized onto food in order that it can be resisted. Mary Douglas argues that the body can represent any bounded system, its boundaries representing the threatened boundaries of the system, its orifices 'its especially vulnerable points' (ibid.: 115, 121). In anorexic ritual the woman is trying to construct and maintain a bounded system, or body, through the exclusion of appetite defined as dangerous and polluting and partially externalized onto food. The mouth is where danger can get in, and the 'bloated' stomach is where the pollution is evident to the anorexic woman and, she believes, to others. But because what is polluting comes from within, resisting it is precarious and contradictory.

Douglas argues that in small persecuted minority groups 'social conditions lend themselves to beliefs which symbolize the body as an imperfect container which can only be made perfect if it can be made impermeable' (ibid.: 158). This is precisely what anorexic women are trying to do, but appetite continually undercuts the impermeable body.

The central anorexic categories are 'safe' and 'dangerous' foods, expressed in the restricted list of foods. All the respondents had a list of specific food and drinks, sometimes as small as one item, that they would allow themselves to eat (see also Wellbourne and Purgold, 1984: 3). Further, they also have a prohibited list – foods and drinks they would rarely, never if they could manage it, eat.

The categories for the most part fall into line with what is currently considered nutritionally good/healthy/wholesome – i.e. fruit and vegetables, bran, wholemeal bread, yoghurt – and bad/un-healthy/'empty' of nutritional value – cakes, sweets, fried foods, fats, fizzy drinks, sugar. As well as the discourse of nutrition, or food as duty, the discourse of diet, or 'slimming' foods, is important in anorexic categorizations – diet coke, low-fat cheeses, crisp-breads, slim soups, skimmed milk, Outline and that staple of all diets, black coffee, all figure prominently. Although reliant on wider social categorizations of food, anorexic categories are both much more rigid, and subject to erratic transformations (Palmer, 1980: 74).

Cultural rules and meanings are transformed in anorexia, and to understand the transformations we must first take a brief look at the dominant cultural meanings of food. Anne Murcott argues that practices and ideas about food should be seen as 'part and parcel of the culture and structure of the societies in which they occur' (Murcott, 1983a: 1). She argues, as we saw above, that cooking and serving food refers to material social relationships, and cites the privileging of men in food distribution as an example. Food and eating, too, have symbolic significance and material and social organization (ibid.: 2–4). She identifies morality as a major symbolic theme in food, suggesting that eating the 'right' food for the 'right' occasion 'conveys a message that the proprieties are being observed' (ibid.: 2).

Paul Atkinson, too, identifies food as a 'code' in which 'cultural oppositions, puzzles and paradoxes may be expressed, and may achieve a symbolic resolution' (Atkinson, 1983: 10). Food and ideas about food convey meanings – including virtue, propriety and nature – and in eating we ingest symbolically as well as concretely, taking in the qualities seen to reside in the food as well as the food itself (ibid.: 10; see also Twigg, 1983: 26). Atkinson analyses 'health foods' to explore the meanings encapsulated in their imagery, finding that 'naturalness' is central. He argues that the main characteristic of health food is that it is seen as natural as opposed to artificial, simple as opposed to adulterated – pure and whole. Health food is healthy because it is natural (Atkinson, 1983: 12–14). Atkinson argues that this imagery is part of a wider ideological strand which contrasts modern urban society with a more 'natural' past – the 'urban pastoral dream' of a past era in which self-sufficiency, personal autonomy and control were possible in a less complicated way of living (ibid.: 15).

Through the expression of 'health' and 'virtue' in the 'natural', our culture expresses an opposition of nature and culture, here through food (ibid.: 12). As Twigg points out, raw food 'in its freshness and newness . . . stands for an uncorrupted reality prior to the distortions and evasions of civilization' (Twigg, 1983: 29). Eating health food, then, allows a resolution at the symbolic level of the pastoral dream and the urban reality. Eating health food equals eating nature, simplicity, wholeness and purity, and gives the sense of personal control which is central to all body-maintenance strategies, as we have seen. We express cultural dissatisfactions in the rejection of 'artificial' food, and resolve the dissatisfaction by eating 'natural' food (Atkinson, 1983: 14–17).

What is healthy about health food is far more, then, than mere 'nutritional' value. In the nature/culture opposition nature is seen as virtuous, and eating natural food is 'a morally desirable act' (ibid.: 16). Eating nature means eating virtue and moral superiority. Eating the unnatural can mean decadent self-indulgence.

Eating as morality versus eating as indulgence is a central opposition in anorexia. One strand of anorexic food categorization is precisely in line with what Atkinson identifies – food as either 'good for you' or 'bad for you' as defined by its degree of healthiness. Anorexic 'safe' food is often health food, but these wider social categories are not simply adopted wholesale by anorexic women. Not all healthy food is safe: Atkinson argues that milk and honey are 'classic' natural foods, conveying purity (ibid.: 11), but whole milk is commonly excluded in anorexia as 'fattening'. Eating health foods in anorexia is the translation of a positive value – taking in nature, health, purity and virtue – into a negative value – *not* taking in pleasure. Here the adulteration of food which is not natural lies more in its attempt to make food more exciting and pleasurable than in the invasion of nature by culture – and it is *this* which anorexic women avoid.

Food in anorexia, then, is separated into two strictly separate categories. 'Safe' food, which is nutritionally valued, low calorie, and not 'fattening', is sanctioned as either doing the body good ('health' foods) or at least not causing any harm ('diet' foods). 'Dangerous' food, food which is off the list, is dangerous because it is food as pure pleasure, which does all harm and no good. The aim is to eat food as fuel:

I wanted foods that were light and didn't fill me up.

(Jane)

They [allowed foods] are crispy and tasty, but light, and do not make me feel heavy and full.

(Sophie)

Here Dally and Gomez's distinction of hunger and appetite is relevant. Dally and Gomez define hunger as a physical response to a disparity between food intake and energy output, and argue that hunger develops 'when physiological changes in the body signal that more fuel is needed . . . [it is] basically concerned with energy balance' (Dally and Gomez, 1980: 14). Appetite, along with habit, determines choice and pleasure in food; it 'dictates what food we fancy or reject . . . appetite anticipates pleasure – from the meal or from the next mouthful' (ibid.: 13). Hunger is a physical appetite, a mental force (ibid.: 14). Hunger is concerned with nutritional requirements, but in appetite food is imbued with symbolic powers and can give symbolic satisfactions: 'Appetite links food with memories and fantasies; with magic and superstition; with love, power and prestige; with happiness and also with misery' (ibid.: 14–17; see also Palmer, 1980: 78–9). It is not only hunger and appetite which motivate us to eat, however:

> Much of our eating depends on habit and routine quite apart from whether we feel hungry. We eat either because everyone else is doing so, or a meal has been prepared at home, or because we are due for a break from work.
>
> (Dally and Gomez, 1980: 22–3)

Dally and Gomez posit hunger as primary, appetite and habit as secondary – appetite and routine are built onto an already existing hunger which has to be satisfied *before* the secondary forces come into play.

Nicky Diamond is critical of the idea of a 'natural hunger mechanism' or 'natural appetite' (Diamond, 1985: 46, 57). She argues that the social structuring of eating *transforms* physical needs and that hunger is 'patterned by social response', gastric juices being produced in accordance with regular food intake and the capacity of the stomach to take in food by regulated amounts. She concludes that 'the experience of "hunger" cannot be freed from meanings, since it is meaning that defines the experience as such' (ibid.: 58). Dally and Gomez see the desire to eat as biological with a social 'overlay' which affects but does not create it; Diamond, on the other hand, argues that hunger, appetite and routine are *all* socially structured.

From the sociological perspective, and bearing in mind our earlier criticisms of sociobiological reasoning, it is the latter perspective which I would argue for. However, I outline the Dally and Gomez position here because it seems to me to be the basis of the widely accepted 'common-sense' view of eating in which hunger equals 'need' and is biological, and appetite equals desire and is social and/or psychological. Further, this common-sense view is worked with in anorexia, where a distinction between hunger as physical need and appetite as desire for pleasure can be detected in the distinction between safe and dangerous foods. Food which can be defined as serving nutritional 'need', empty of pleasure is (at first) allowable; food which socially or personally is defined as pleasurable and 'empty' of nutritional value must be eliminated.

Although the specific categorizations are to an extent subject to transformations dependent on individual biography (cf. Palmer, 1980: 23; Atkinson, 1983: 11), there is a great deal of similarity in anorexic women's allowed lists. I asked the women what they ate, and why they chose those particular foods: Fiona eats fruit, wholemeal bread and '"Light" Philadelphia cheese (in limitation)', black and decaffinated tea and coffee and mineral water; 'The fruit makes me feel clean and fresh and so do the drinks. The bread and cheese are consumed to keep my parents happy.'

> I eat more or less the same each day . . .2 tablespoons yoghurt and banana, 2 crispbreads and tomato, lettuce, 2 tablespoons cottage cheese, apple, cornflakes.
>
> (Laura)

> even now as I recover . . . I tend to stick to low calorie food and drinks. I eat bran, oats, vegetables, fruits and things that I can calorie count . . . at my worst I ate one Farley's rusk per day for weeks. As I declined I ate All Bran, cottage cheese, meat, fish and vegetables . . . I know they are low calorie foods, I know how to keep charge of my weight. It means that they take longer to eat and make me feel full. I feel better about eating them as I don't feel guilty.
>
> (Anne)

Tracy eats low calorie foods and drinks, salad and fruit: 'I don't feel so threatened by the prospect of eating food, if it is low in calories.' Lynne eats bread, cheese, yoghurt, fruit, coffee, tea and pasta:

> It has nothing to do with taste. It is just I know their calorie content and feel safe with these foods. There are loads of things I have never tried, I wouldn't feel safe with them . . . they feel like unknown territory.

I asked the women to describe what they would eat in a typical day if they kept to plan, and how they would then feel:

> Breakfast – coffee
> Lunch – 1 sachet slim soup, 1 small apple
> Supper – 1 sachet slim soup, 1 chinese leaf (1 oz.)
> Evening – 1 Shape yoghurt
> Bed – 1 small apple
> (Sundays: 1 slice toast for supper instead of soup)
> Relieved and calm but hungry . . . I stick to a rigid timetable and panic if I am out and can't eat at exact times.
>
> (Patricia)

Sharon eats 2 meals daily, either one meal of All Bran, fruit and yoghurt and one of vegetables, or two of vegetables: 'I rarely, if ever, eat what I've not planned.'

> 1 Weetabix and ¼ pint skimmed milk, 1 low-fat yoghurt and apple, 5 oz. jacket potato and bowl of salad.
> On a high.
>
> (Margaret)

I eat the same food every day and I drink the same drink, no change, except if I am having a binge:

> Daily: 5 tins Diet Coca Cola
>   4 apples
>   2 oranges
>   8 Crispbread with Shape cheese
>   3 black coffees
>   Sometimes 1 bowl of bran with water.

> I like these foods and drinks because they are not fattening and do not have any carbohydrate in them and above all they feel safe to me.
>
> (Karen)

I asked what food the women rarely or never ate, and why this should be so: Sarah never eats full-fat milk, oranges, tuna, cheese, butter, bread, cakes: 'They make me frightened – that I've done something *wrong* eating them – "forbidden" foods to mother and sister. They see it as a *sin* to eat them and instant fatness.' Sharon never eats fats, meat, fried food, carbohydrates, sweet things or alcohol: 'I feel that they're unhealthy (I know that carbohydrates such as bread and rice aren't – but I avoid eating them.' Tracy never eats milk, cakes or sweets: 'I feel threatened. I feel they will make me fat.'

The allowed foods require minimal or usually no cooking, and very little preparation. Karen eats cottage cheese and apples because 'I like the taste of cottage cheese and apples plus they are low calories and come in small sizes.' One reason for cooking is to enhance the pleasure of eating; here food is the result of creative labour and, as we have seen, is intended to produce pleasure for others and expresses women's role as domestic servicers. Pleasure in eating being precisely what the anorexic is trying to eliminate, preparation and cooking are excluded from anorexic eating.

I asked if the women had *favourite* foods, and if so, did they eat them? Beatrice's favourites are hard cheese, grapes and milky coffee; grapes are a 'safe' food, coffee sometimes allowable; cheese is the real danger:

> I'm careful with hard cheese – eat it just on Friday and Sunday evening when I'm at my mother-in-law's as if I have it in my home I'd never be able to leave it alone until I'd eaten the lot. I allow myself a treat on these days and feel 'safe'.

> Toast and marmalade. Roast meat and roast potatoes. Fruit crumble. Greek yoghurt. Chips. Once a year, at Christmas, I have meat. Once a week I have a piece of toast. The rest – never.
> (Patricia)

Even after women feel they have recovered from anorexia (in so far as they see recovery as possible), they still restrict their favourite foods strictly.[2] Anne now eats some of the food she likes but never eats desserts; Sarah eats her favourites – eggs, butter and cheese – 'all the time . . . 3 times a week . . . [and] once a week' respectively.

Food that gives pleasure is dangerous food; the aim is to eliminate the pleasure, and eventually the food itself: Alicia never eats biscuits, cake, crisps, alcohol, fried food, cereals and chocolate:

I have completely got out of the habit – I cut them out of my diet years ago and now refuse them automatically. I'm also petrified of eating too much carbohydrate.

At first I wouldn't allow myself to enjoy food, but then it really did become sickening and abhorrent. I can't remember what I enjoyed before I was ill.

(Jane)

I have got to the point where I have no favourite foods.

(Zoe)

I'm not sure what a hungry feeling is any more.

(Verity)

Annette never eats 'milk . . . and most food; I never ever fancy them. I never seem to feel like anything.'
The safe category contracts as the dangerous category expands; the hunger/appetite distinction loses its force as the category of forbidden food expands to take in all food.[3] The ultimate aim, usually unfulfillable, is to eat nothing at all:

Before, I was pleased [if she ate to plan] but must make more effort to eat less and look for ways to cut down and this I did gradually by reducing meals and then cutting them out one by one.

(Anne)

I asked the women what they would do if they could eat nothing at all and yet stay healthy – would they do so, and how would this feel?

Yes – wonderful!!!

(Zoe)

Yes. Clean.

(Celia)

Yes – fantastic – so alive, healthy and clean.

(Fiona)

Yes. It would have felt a great relief and freedom.

(Jane)

Yes, this would be the answer to my dreams! I feel elated even now just thinking about it. I really feel my body does not need

food and can function on what I allow it . . . I wouldn't eat even
if I didn't put weight on. There is nothing I would crave to eat!

(Annette)

I would love to abolish food and eating and yet stay healthy. I
would feel in control and not guilty.

(Paula)

It would be the best solution to the problem, no more worrying
about weight or calories or food at all. When I starve myself I
always want to continue as long as possible.

(Barbara)

Yes. I always look forward to the time when energy can be
obtained through tablets of a certain calorie-value thus avoiding
any contact with food or cooking and planning food.

(Andrea)

In reality, the nearest the anorexic woman can get to this ultimate
state is to get her intake of food, and consequently her weight, as
low as possible. In this closest approximation, she feels wonderful:

elated and triumphant

(Patricia)

such an ego-booster! . . . happy, proud, feel successful, feel
completely in charge of everything

(Frances)

GREAT . . . thin and clean at 4 stone 13 lb.

(Celia)

elated and very triumphant . . . my blood pressure is high which
gives me headaches but I feel fine.

(Annette)

Most anorexic women do eat, at least a little, and cope with the
anxiety of eating in a variety of ways. Some get rid of the food as
soon as possible. Marie exercises after eating, to 'burn up' the food,
Annette while eating minimized her panic by working out how
many laxatives she would need to take, and what was the best thing
to take them with, in order to get the food out of her body, and
Hannah writes:

Before I eat (or ate) I felt afraid that I had held out too long;
while eating my main idea was how I could get rid of the food

in one way or another – and this thought filled my head until I felt empty again.

Una explains that while bingeing she felt that she must keep eating until she could vomit; if she didn't she was 'obsessed with the idea of the food being absorbed by my body'. Sheila writes that: 'I just regurgitate stuff sometimes and spit it out without chewing. What is regurgitated goes in fads/cycles. At present it is peanuts and "Lion" bars.' When Frances has food in her stomach she is really frightened: 'it has to be got rid of as soon as possible'.

For the women who don't or can't bring themselves to purge or vomit, and in cases where what is eaten is the allowed daily minimum, food that stays in the body is hemmed in and controlled through a ritualized eating pattern. The most common ritual which emerged from the survey was eating exactly the same foods, in the same amount, in the same order and usually at the same time and in the same place every day:

> Every day I eat exactly the same food and exactly the same amount. [I] eat exactly the same amount of crispbread and . . . cut the same amount of cheese to put on the crispbread.
>
> (Eve)

> I break certain shapes of crispbread, etc. off to eat. I arrange my food (which is the same every day) in the same way on the plate, and eat it in the same order, at exactly the same time.
>
> (Sophie)

> Eating at a set time, in the same place and exactly the same food each day.
>
> (Margaret)

> My eating pattern is so rigid and controlled. I don't *consciously* plan, but I automatically eat virtually the same food each day.
>
> (Polly)

Similarly, Wellbourne and Purgold quote 'Della': 'Barriers of time lock in on you. Clench you in their iron fists. You cannot eat if it is not the right time – exactly' (Wellbourne and Purgold, 1984: 25).

Controlling the anxiety by 'thought-rituals' also featured:

I always keep recalling it [her plan] to my mind just to check I haven't eaten anything I might have forgotten.

(Lynne)

I organize my eating as the day unfolds; counting calories after every mouthful and giving myself a calorie intake for each day . . . I have to keep a constant watch on my eating during all hours that I'm awake. I'm often too exhausted to feel any sense of achievement until the following day when I can look back and think: 'Yesterday was a "GOOD" day.'

(Andrea)

'Staple' foods . . . somehow they seem safe. There was a time I would mentally break down everything I ate into the equivalent 'staples' – calculating if I'd just eaten more or less than if I'd had, say, my usual bowl of muesli, or piece of bread and cheese.

(Irene)

The actual process of eating is also ritualized; food is separated into tiny and precise quantities, eaten in small mouthfuls, chewed with extreme thoroughness or timed:

I cut my Ryvitas up into 5 bits each slice. Each bit lasts while I read one page on a book. I then eat my vegetables followed by fruit. I only eat in bed.

(Beatrice)

I eat by the clock – still very much the same type of food for each meal.

(Laura)

I tend to eat things in exactly [the] same order and I do cut up bread into fingers. I have to have the same plates, cup and cutlery.

(Alicia)

I used to have to eat at set times and cut my apple in quarters, then take each piece and cut paper thin slices to eat as slowly as possible.

(Carol)

Celia chews every mouthful seven times, Yvonne cuts her food into tiny portions and pushes it around her plate, and Sarah eats 'tiny mouthfuls' and chews her food 'to an absolute pulp'. Jane writes:

I would cut food into very small pieces, take very small mouthfuls, and take a very long time chewing. I used to time how long it took to eat certain things, e.g. a pot of yoghurt, then I had to keep to these times.

The 'point' of this behaviour, I would argue, is two-fold. First, as we have seen, food for the anorexic woman is dangerous, and its principal meanings centre around the chaos and insatiability of appetite. Rituals of content, time, place and method, therefore, impose order on potential chaos and act to contain its threat. Second the rituals postpone the actual act of swallowing the food; they make eating unlike 'ordinary' eating since ingestion is allowable only as part of a ritualized pattern which encompasses the total environment of the 'meal', not just the act of swallowing itself. The ultimate aim is not to swallow at all, and as close as possible an approximation to this is the aim of the ritualized eating pattern. Sometimes it can come very close:

[I] would feel as if I was going to vomit. Sometimes I would have to force myself to swallow after chewing the food for a long time.
(Marie)

Anorexic eating rituals, then, connect not only to the direct act of swallowing but to the total 'food situation', as Polly and Sharon explain:

They've [her rituals] varied over the years – but they apply both to my surroundings when I eat [e.g. clean, warm, comfortable, etc.] and to the actual food [e.g. biscuits whole not broken; cheese cut into neat slices, everything 'perfect']. I try to keep these rituals to a minimum, even to the extent of deliberately not washing my hands! – because they are a nightmare.

I do cut food into very small pieces. I always wash up any dirty dishes and pots [used in preparation] before I've eaten. Also, I like to drink a large glass of diluted fruit juice while I eat – it can take up to 45 minutes for me to complete eating a one-course meal. I almost always have a cup of coffee once I've cleared away all the utensils.

Getting herself ready for the day also formed part of Irene's rituals: 'I did have other "rituals" though – silly things like the way I dressed, or the order I'd do things when I got up in the morning.' As we've seen, exercise after eating figures in anorexia, and many

anorexic women also weigh themselves frequently, often daily, and
sometimes more: Paula weighs herself every two hours, Yvonne
twelve times daily.

Although food, weight and eating are the principal areas of
anorexic ritualized control, the body as a whole is treated, I would
argue, as a 'protected zone'. I am indebted to Caroline O'Toole of
Glasgow Anorexic Aid for her suggestion that I ask women for
their feelings about sexuality – which is a common feature of the
literature on anorexia – and also about physical intimacy/touching
as a whole. Caroline feels that many, probably most, anorexic
women not only avoid sex but prefer not to be touched at all. The
avoidance of sex is borne out by the literature (e.g. Anderson,
1977: 14; Hsu, 1980: 1044), and also by the responses to the
survey, which suggested also that anorexic women prefer not to
be touched at all, and to have 'space' around their bodies. Out of
the 35 women 30 either disliked or feared sex, or described
themselves as having no sexual feelings during the anorexia:

> I was very afraid of sex and thought of it as something bad and
> wrong.
>
> (Jane)

> [I] used to split off from myself during sex with my husband,
> couldn't be both a good little girl and a mistress at the same time.
>
> (Marie)

> I have become very cold and hate being touched, I have no
> sexual desires.
>
> (Sandra)

> [Anorexia] completely numbs those feelings.
>
> (Anne)

Some explicitly categorized sex as heterosexual, some talked in the
abstract, and none defined sex as involving other women.

With only six exceptions the women either disliked or feared
non-sexual touching too:

> I feel threatened, sometimes almost claustrophobic.
>
> (Irene)

> I cannot cope with anyone coming close or touching me even if
> someone touches me on the shoulders or back, the emotional

pain hurts, I cringe so much I want to curl into a ball and hide,
I feel like barbed wire.

(Eve)

Some women saw their avoidance of physical contact as imposed
on them by the illness, and wrote poignantly of their wish that they
could let people get close to them:

I resent people being physically close to me, but I yearn for one
special person to hold me and comfort me.

(Frances)

I like space around me. I used to be a very cuddly person and
hate being so detached.

(Norma)

If the elimination of physical pleasure is the central aim of anorexia, and the body is created at the symbolic level as need-less and
inviolable, then physical detachment is necessary. In anorexia
eating and food become symbolic of all desires and their objects.
Desire as a whole is crystallized into the desire for food, the arena
in which satisfaction/fulfillment of desire is most possible for
women.

The ultimate aim and purpose of anorexia is the denial of
appetite, and at the height of anorexia, when the illness can still
be seen in a wholly positive light, denial itself equals pleasure,
achievement, mastery and virtue, with hunger the internal and
emaciation the external 'signs' of that denial (cf. Palmer, 1980: 21):

If I didn't eat I felt very high and full of energy, very proud of
myself for having self control.

(Marie)

Absolutely great – a huge sense of achievement.

(Fiona)

I feel completely happy, confident, able to go out and talk to
people – I feel in total control. I feel as if I have achieved
something.

(Eve)

I do so less and less [eat] because the vague sense of satisfaction
is both short-lived and far-outweighed, when faced with fat and

food or a sense of virtue and tautness and no food . . . it's a fairly easy choice.

(Sheila)

Wellbourne and Purgold argue that it is this sense of achievement which explains why anorexic women keep on and on losing weight long after the original target weight has been reached. Losing weight comes to mean control, success and competence, and weight gain means failure. Consequently, the 'target' gets progressively lower (Wellbourne and Purgold, 1984: 31). This, then, is the 'moral spiral' of anorexia.

DANGER

In spite of what one reads in the psychiatric literature of anorexic stubborn invincibility, the anorexic woman's 'wilful and covertly triumphant pursuit of thinness' (Casper *et al*, 1980: 1030), the denial and control of anorexic ritualized eating, which gives such a sense of safety, power and virtue, is, in fact, infinitely precarious. It is only ever achieved temporarily and, even when on an anorexic high, the anorexic woman feels the threat of insatiability, danger and chaos lurking around her. The threats to her control are two-fold but of far from equal value. I'd like to take a brief look at the subsidiary threat – the interference of other people – before going on to concentrate on hunger itself as the principal harbinger of doom. The threat of control by others will also figure in the discussion of the anorexic woman's perception of herself as the object of medical control; her sense of control by parents, friends and social values in general *before* the onset of the illness has been discussed above. It is this sense of persecution, coupled with the function of anorexic ritual in excluding disorder, rather than 'retarded cognition' or 'limited thinking' which make the anorexic woman stick rigidly to her eating pattern (Crisp and Fransella, 1972: 405).

Anorexic women are immensely anxious about situations in which they have to eat with other people, or, even worse, have to eat a meal someone else has prepared:

If I have to go out and eat more than my 'ration' I feel very depressed, fat, miserable and resentful . . . to keep my friends I have to eat normal meals at least once in ten days. That is a great source of conflict and resentment, and is an area where I feel I am out of control, though I attempt to control how much they give me and what.

(Patricia)

Sometimes I can't stand eating (especially if forced to eat something because it's sociable to eat different courses in someone's home).

(Andrea)

I have a husband who has to be deceived in order for life to carry on peacefully; [she would be completely in control of her eating] but people try to interfere.

(Annette)

When asked if she would give up eating entirely if it were possible, and how this would feel, Margaret replied: 'Yes – terrific as there would be no pressure on me by others to eat for my health's sake.'

Other people, then, are perceived by anorexic women as a threat to their control of food; what is seen as concern by family and friends is seen as interference by anorexic women. As Wellbourne and Purgold point out, the intervention of others is experienced by anorexic women as 'assaults on anorexic integrity' (Wellbourne and Purgold, 1984: 96). The principal threat to the control of food intake is, however, appetite itself. Wellbourne and Purgold argue thus:

the sufferers feel that if their control slipped just once and they ate food not sanctioned by their private rule-book they would 'lose control' or 'go to pieces'.

(ibid.: 3)

They live, then, 'in a state of constant anxiety lest a momentary loss of control may lead to . . . disintegration' (ibid.: 94). And it is in this context that the 'tricks' and deceptions of anorexia (Dexter, 1980: 326–7) are meaningful.

Only six of the women who replied to the survey felt that they were totally in control of their eating. Every 'meal' is an ordeal; fear and ambivalence are its characteristics:

[When eating I am] sometimes extremely panicky (always take the phone off so I can get through the ordeal). Other times I feel desperate and eat too fast and fill up quickly. I think about food from the moment I wake at 5.30–6 a.m. until bedtime at about 11. I am anxious to eat and basically enjoy the tastes when

I'm eating but often get very full and feel I shouldn't have eaten
it.

(Sandra)

Tense, guilty, frightened of retribution and disease . . . I look
forward to eating, though with apprehension. While I'm actually eating I usually feel good about the food at first, and about
the nourishment it's giving me. But gradually as I eat, guilt takes
over, and I feel over-indulgent, bloated and miserable.

(Polly)

Tremendous tension, should I, shouldn't I, very guilty at every
mouthful. No sense of enjoyment at all.

(Lynne)

I usually wind up thinking, 'I love this, I hate this, why am I
doing this?' and stop then and there.

(Sheila)

Sheila adds that before she eats she feels 'frantic for food', while
eating she feels simultaneous satisfaction and guilt, and afterwards
'remorse and panic'. Sarah writes that before she eats she feels
'something like terror – it feels like it is doing the wrong thing
eating it and wanting it'. Each day represents a 'battle' with food
in which eating is staved off until the evening. The struggle is
between the terror of eating and the pleasure of food, of giving
herself 'what I wanted and needed'.

Eve also expresses the struggle between *needing* food, which can
be acceptable, and *wanting* to eat, which isn't:

Before I eat anything I always contemplate whether I really
need to eat it because I feel so good when I am empty. During
eating food I always feel guilty and think about how many
calories the food I am eating contains. After I have eaten I
always worry and say to myself 'maybe I have eaten too much'.

Any pleasure that remains is, as Norma writes, 'soon spoilt by guilt,
was I eating too much . . . would I stop eating?'

No matter how small the amount, and how rigidly controlled
the eating is, anxiety remains. Asked how she feels when eating to
plan, Verity writes that she feels 'in control but still dissatisfied,
leading on so you keep cutting down, looking for the day when
being thin is going to make you happy'. The plan does not in itself

represent sufficient security, and keeping to it is in any case difficult:

> I feel angry with myself because most times I haven't intended to eat and then I find myself eating something.
>
> (Fiona)

> If it's my 'safe' foods OK. If not – my heart's beating ten to the dozen and I feel panic-stricken – unless I'm having a binge and know I'm going to get rid of it later – but while I'm eating I'm telling myself what a disgusting pig I am and wonder what damage I'm doing to my health.
>
> (Beatrice)

> I lose control regularly despite all my efforts to combat it.
>
> (Andrea)

Having 'given in' to extra-plan eating, the danger of the loss of control can be symbolically contained by some by getting the food out of the mouth as soon as possible:

> Sometimes I swallow quickly just to get it over and done with.
>
> (Irene)

> I want to swallow it to get it out of the way.
>
> (Lynne)

> It's something I've got to swallow as fast as possible.
>
> (Margaret)

More typically, however, this is no real solution; even if the food can no longer be tasted in the mouth it is still felt in the stomach; almost all the women reported feeling simultaneously over-full *and* hungry after eating. The almost inevitable choice of word to describe this feeling is 'bloated'. Being bloated is both an internal sign of over-indulgence to the anorexic woman and, it is thought, a very obvious external sign to other people. The guilt and depression that the anorexic woman has 'over-eaten' can become unbearable; some women take steps to get rid of the evidence. I asked the women how they felt with food in their stomachs, and how they dealt with their feelings: Margaret's 'solution' is no solution at all:

> Guilty and that I've to remove it by some means or other as quick as I can.

I feel about 9 months pregnant. My stomach feels so bloated I think that people must notice. Therefore I have to get it out as soon as possible!

(Annette)

I feel when I've eaten that I look fat and bloated and want to get rid of the feeling by taking laxatives, etc.

(Sandra)

Sometimes if I feel too bloated I make myself sick.

(Eve)

I used to feel guilty, bloated, obsessed by the food I had absorbed, longing for it to go. I felt better when I was empty.

(Norma)

Bloated. Worried that I might gain weight. Feel a lack of control. Sometimes the feeling is so intolerable I have to go and vomit, though this usually only happens when I have eaten more than just fresh fruit and vegetables.

(Paula)

The act of eating is the arena in which the precarious nature of anorexic control is most directly experienced. Rigid planning and the ritualizations which surround eating serve to create a partial control which alleviates but only rarely contains hunger. The fear of a chaos of appetite is the context in which anorexic food control is meaningful; Paula when eating feels: 'worried that I might gain weight and worried that having started to eat, I may be unable to stop'. Norma writes that when she managed to eat to plan: 'I remember feeling great temporarily [mentally] but still hungry, and terrified of *having* to eat more, to let go and eat.' The fear of insatiability surrounds eating. Sophie fears 'that it will go totally out of control, and I will not be able to stop'. And Lynne writes

I feel if I let go of my controls, anarchy would set in, and my body would rebel. Would I suddenly turn into a 10-stone animal? . . .What I worry about, is the 'full' feeling, when you ought to know you have had enough food, I don't seem to be able to recognize that feeling. So I feel if I started to eat when would I stop?

Norton quotes a patient saying much the same thing: 'If ever I've been forced to eat anything on my plate, I feel myself getting bigger and bigger, expanding like a balloon' (Norton, 1983: 312).

The loss of control which so terrifies anorexic women centres around eating and getting 'fat', but it can be extended to cover other areas of their lives:

> I felt that if I let go the control, then everything would fall apart and be chaotic, and I would be completely overwhelmed by it all.
>
> (Jane)

Marie feels that if she gave up trying to control her eating, 'I wouldn't be in control of anything then.'

> If I broke that control, would self-control in other areas go also? I felt it would and therefore clung to control over food.
>
> (Hannah)

The denial of first pleasure and subsequently appetite itself which is the ultimate aim of anorexia, can give intense satisfaction but is highly precarious. I found little evidence of what Casper *et al.* describe as the anorexic woman's 'unusual ability to suppress or tolerate hunger feelings' (Casper *et al.*, 1980: 1030). Again this would seem to be a case of psychiatry taking for granted as true what is part of the anorexic defence against psychiatric intervention. The anorexic control envied by others and struggled over in the psychiatric encounter is maintained only with extreme difficulty and in a context of constant setbacks. Falling into chaos is both a real experience and a psychic terror. It is to this annihilation of control that we now turn.

CHAOS

Twenty-five of the women said that they used to, or still did binge. Only one, however, described herself as bulimic. For the others, bingeing is part of anorexia, the other side of the coin of control, what makes it necessary, and what endangers it.

Psychiatric opinion is divided on whether bulimia and anorexia should be considered 'different entities' (Anderson, 1977; Chiodo and Latimer, 1983), whether they are essentially the same disorder (Wellbourne and Purgold, 1984: 2) or whether bulimia is a 'subgroup' of anorexia (Casper *et al.*, 1980: 1030; Garfinkel *et al.*, 1980).

Casper *et al*. set the scene for the debate by arguing that:

> the occurrence of bulimia (rapid consumption of large amounts
> of food in a short period of time) is a perplexing phenomenon,
> because its presence contradicts the common belief that patients
> with anorexia are always firm in their abstinence from food.
>
> (ibid.: 1030)

In their study, 47 per cent of the respondents admitted to bingeing, and they suggest that while bulimia was neglected in the
older psychiatric literature, 'those who looked for it have generally
found it' (ibid.: 1031, 1034; see also Morgan, Purgold and Wellbourne, 1983). Casper *et al*. argue that 'bulimics' can be
distinguished from 'fasting patients' chiefly by a stronger appetite
and a lesser capacity to tolerate hunger, which lead to 'impaired
control' in eating and in their lives in general (ibid.: 1034, 1030–4).
However, they are further distinguished by being older, more
'extrovert', suffering more depression, anxiety, guilt and obsession
with food (ibid.: 1031–5). They argue that bulimia is associated
with a longer illness, repeated hospitalizations, and 'a less successful social adjustment' (ibid.: 1034).

These findings lead Casper *et al*. to hypothesize that bulimia
may be 'a sign of chronicity', or, that to become bulimic the patient
may need greater 'physiological and psychological maturity', or,
and this is the preferred thesis, that bulimia may represent 'a more
serious psychopathology' (ibid.: 1034–5). They argue that for these
more disturbed women, bingeing is 'emotionally soothing' (ibid.:
1034), and, followed by vomiting, forms: 'a complex defensive
manoeuvre in which food is abnormally employed to relieve
profoundly disturbing impulses, feelings, and thoughts' (ibid.:
1035). This analysis is remarkable for its mixture of perspicacity
and obfuscation. Initially Casper *et al*. sense that the presence of a
significant amount of binge/vomiting in patients defined as anorexic threatens the idea that anorexia involves a transcendence
of appetite. This insight *could* lead to a recognition that anorexia
is rarely, and then only temporarily, a transcendence of appetite,
and is more correctly seen as an extended struggle *with* appetite,
in which the ritualized control of eating is the weapon and hunger
the enemy. And in arguing that 'fasters' cherish hunger and obtain
from it 'a sense of mastery' they come close to recognizing that
anorexia is far from easy and 'triumphant' but is in fact a desperate
struggle with a powerful internal enemy (ibid.: 1034, 1030). In-

stead, however, the old answer of a particular psychopathology explains that while 'fasting patients' *can* 'suppress' 'deny' 'ignore' or 'tolerate' appetite – in short, transcend it – the especially disturbed and unsuccessfully adjusted bulimic is 'just' a failed anorexic.

Similarly, although they note that bulimics have been ill longer and hospitalized more often, the explanation of bulimia as a development of anorexia is given short shrift. Although they point out that whether or not the women binge, they still experience 'a similar perpetual fear of not being able to stop eating' (ibid.: 1034) this does not lead them to see the fear of insatiability and the fantasy of bingeing as just as important as the actual binge.

This point is taken up by Wellbourne and Purgold, who argue that what defines anorexia is a characteristic way of *thinking*, in which fear of weight gain, and control of weight, rather than emaciation, are central (Wellbourne and Purgold, 1984: 25–9). They argue thus that bulimics are anorexics, that there are 'no characteristic bulimic ideas' (ibid.: 6). All anorexics, as they point out, are interested in food, and feel that their appetite is 'too powerful', 'insatiable and demanding' and 'must at all costs be curbed' (ibid.: 3). This 'anorexic thinking' can lead to either starvation or binge/vomiting and 'effectiveness' is the only real difference (ibid.: 6).

The fear of bingeing was an ever-present worry to the women in the survey, and I would argue that it is this which inspires anorexic control. The reality of bulimia could more plausibly be explained by the realization that the immense difficulty of main-taining anorexic control means that the longer the illness, the more likely it is that control will periodically slip (see Palmer, 1980: 29). And since control of appetite is the central aim of anorexia, it is not surprising that depression, anxiety and guilt accompany its loss.

Furthermore, if we look at psychiatric intervention from the anorexic perspective, we can argue that bulimia could well be a response to the disruption of control which hospitalization entails. Bulimia, defined as bingeing *and* vomiting, is better seen as an expression of the 'disturbing impulses' of controlled appetite than relief of those impulses. The idea that women who binge experi-ence stronger hunger than those who do not is based on the women's response to psychiatric questioning and does not con-sider how careful women must be about what they feel able to reveal to such questioners. Denial of hunger is, of course, one of the main anorexic strategies in maintaining control when other people intervene in their eating. Further, the argument that bulimics suffer from 'impaired control' contradicts the argument that they are naturally hungrier – is it that they have less control or is what they are trying to control stronger?

In the discussion and analysis of anorexic women's descriptions of bingeing which follows I hope, then, to show that the binge as an ever-present threat to anorexic control is a central feature of anorexia, in which the fear of insatiability which necessitates that control becomes a reality. While the question of how much women actually eat in a binge is, as we saw in Chapter 4, experientially significant for women, it is not, I would argue, an element which meaningfully distinguishes groups of anorexic women. Rather, it is the *meaning* of the binge, however large or small it is, which is important.

I asked the women whether they ate different foods during a binge, and, if so, how they would explain their choice:

I drink fruit squash. I eat mostly sweet things, sometimes crisps and occasionally I'll cook some meat but not often. Usually it's marmalade out of the jar (about ¾ lb.), mincemeat (1 lb.), 2 litres ice-cream,½ packet biscuits,½ cake,½ lb. cheese, ¾ lb. pickle, a Swiss roll – this would be fairly typical. Sometimes I vomit and return to the kitchen again.

(Paula)

I drink gallons of milkshake, I eat ice-cream, cakes, pastries, pork pies, chips, sweets, chocolates, bread, roast potatoes. I can eat half a loaf of bread, 15 fish fingers, 6 fried eggs, 2 platefuls of chips, 4 doughnuts, 6 chocolate cakes, 2 large bars of chocolate, 10 bars of Mars bar, etc., 1 litre of ice-cream, and probably more. Because they are foods I forbid myself on my days of dieting.

(Tracy)

for me a binge usually consists of: 4 caramel chocolate bars, liquorice toffees, cream cakes,½ loaf of bread. Because these foods are really naughty – full of fat and I never allow myself these things, so if I binge I might as well lose control and eat all the worst things possible.

(Eve)

Binge foods – muesli, whole milk, butter and sugar mixed together, jam, raisins, orange juice, bread and butter – something to do with them being forbidden, 'naughty' – in a desperate attempt to be nicer to myself – to make up for something, someone – possibly my mother . . . for not being accepted as my own person as I am.

(Sarah)

All but one of the women who binged ate mostly, although not exclusively, carbohydrates and sweet things (see Boskind-Lodahl, 1976: 351–2). The main explanation given for this was that these are 'forbidden' foods the rest of the time, but the accepted psychiatric explanation of a purely physical craving was expressed by two of the women:

I think it is because I crave these foods and yet forbid myself to eat them.

(Fiona)

before a binge I would have a deep craving (like an addiction) and I felt I just had to eat them.

(Karen)

Practicalities also intrude in the choice of binge foods; Frances explains her choice of foods as being 'easy to eat/swallow and when mixed with enough fluid, are easy to bring back up'. Barbara's explanation also centres on convenience: 'They're always convenient, easy to eat and read, or eat and watch TV. Can take them to my room. Quick to prepare, no cooking involved.'

The choice of food that needs cooking, or any amount of preparation is as rare in binges as in the anorexic plan. Barbara's explanation reveals a further, central facet of binges: in spite of the fact that forbidden and pleasure-laden foods are being eaten, the attention is directed *away* from the taste of the food. As Palmer argues, in a binge food is eaten 'rapidly and avidly but with little pleasure' (Palmer, 1980: 26).

I asked the women if they ate in a different way when bingeing:

All the food is laid out and I just attack it; tearing at the packaging like an animal. My hands are working all the time to get handfuls of food into my mouth, working systematically through everything until I just cannot eat another thing.

(Carol)

In a mad panic to stuff the food down me as quickly as possible, hardly tasting or chewing it.

(Fiona)

Yes I used to eat without even noticing I was doing it – my eyes fixed on the TV or staring into space. I used to eat so messily too that it would make me furious with myself.

(Una)

I feel like an animal, dipping in with my fingers or tipping the carrots into my mouth. I usually crouch down by the fridge to do this.

(Sandra)

When I feel a binge coming on I feel so tense I eat anything without even tasting it, at very high speed, towards the end of the binge I am usually just throwing the food into my mouth and even into my face with such speed that sometimes I swallow things whole, uncooked, frozen.

(Eve)

I *never* use knife and fork and a plate at the table – just a spoon and my hands. I certainly eat very fast and hardly chew it, just swallow it.

(Paula)

Like a maniac that hasn't eaten in years! I ram one food after another into my mouth, hardly having time to butter the next slice of bread beforehand.

(Tracy)

The main characteristics of binge eating which emerged from the survey, then, were *speed*, *animalistic manner* and a sense of *compulsion*. The women ate as fast as they possibly could, in a manner they describe as irrational, usually animalistic – 'like a scavenging animal' (Sophie), 'like a wolf' (Una) – and with compulsion but not pleasure – 'I eat quickly almost in a panic – don't really taste it' (Laura), '[I] cannot stop' (Sophie). Although they are giving themselves what is usually denied them, indulgence, I would argue, does not equal pleasure. Rather, they fear being at the mercy of their appetite, which they feel unable to control. The binge is unstoppable; it ends only when the food runs out. Cooking, preparation, laying the table and relishing the meal are all conspicuous by their absence. The opposite of denial in anorexia is compulsion and chaos, not pleasure.

Boskind-Lodahl argues that women gain pleasure from being out of control in the binge, and that shame and guilt come afterwards (Boskind-Lodahl, 1976: 351–2). She argues:

> the binge brings about a union between the mind and the body. One gives one's self to the food, to the moment completely. There is a complete loss of control (ego). It is an absolute here-and-now experience, a kind of ecstasy.
>
> (ibid.: 352)

I would suggest that, far from union and ecstasy the binge means failure and surrender. Anorexia is an attempt to *create* a self, or ego, out of the control of need; in the binge control is swallowed up and destroyed by appetite. Boskind-Lodahl argues that 'bulimarexic' women are involved 'in a struggle against a part of the self rather than a struggle towards a self' (ibid.: 352), and implies that the 'unification' of the two 'halves' in the binge is therefore pleasurable. I would argue that unity is impossible for anorexic women; either the controlling ego or the insatiable flesh can dominate, but they cannot be integrated, since the dominance of the former over the latter is the point of anorexic control.

Boskind-Lodahl implies, Leslie Swartz argues, that the 'pleasure' of the binge comes from 'the woman's "natural" wish to be in tune with her body's desires'. Boskind-Lodahl suggests that 'the body is "correct" in its desires whereas the mind is warped' in trying to block 'the forces of nature' (Swartz, 1985: 431). Similarly, Orbach and Eichenbaum see bingeing as an assertion of 'natural' desires and argue that the bingeing 'part' of the anorexic woman is the part therapists can work with in the return to normality (ibid.: 431; Orbach and Eichenbaum, 1983: 90). This biologistic prioritizing is irrelevant if one sees both mind and body as socially created. The anorexic woman while bingeing is not surrendering to 'nature' – unquestionably good and virtuous – but to an appetite which both she and her culture define as dangerous and disgusting.

What bingeing in its extremity reveals is an insatiability which the anorexic feels to be ever-present danger. Wellbourne and Purgold's 'Della' writes that:

> breaking out of control, out of the order means no order. To

break out of the strictly-imposed regulations means one has no limits. It means that one will move to the extremes of human indulgence.

(Wellbourne and Purgold, 1984: 25)

The binge is a furtive business conducted in solitude; the terrifying possibility of being 'caught in the act' of insatiability is removed as far as possible: 'I had to be alone in a room with the curtains closed so that no one could possibly see me' (Paula). But *any* eating has the character of a guilty and secret activity (see also Dally and Gomez, 1980: 17). Out of the 35 respondents, 31 preferred to eat alone if at all possible. Beatrice only eats at night, in bed, 'away from others'; Annette writes that 'no-one must see me swallow' – before she eats she worries 'in case anyone catches me'. Fiona writes:

> I find now that I can only force myself to eat in the presence of my parents but I hate this and if I see them watching me eat, I stop immediately and become embarrassed. I cannot, however, eat in front of other members of my family or in front of my friends.

With food inside them anorexic women feel: 'afraid, dirty and weak' (Karen); 'bloated, guilty, greedy and a failure' (Una); 'greedy and as though I am guilty of some misdeed' (Fiona). When they are alone, this is bad enough. In front of others it is insupportable:

> [Eating] in front of my family: *guilty – bad.*
>
> (Sarah)

> When I eat and have food in my mouth I feel dirty, guilty and fat. If someone is present – which I cannot help sometimes – my mouth feels as if it is numb and paralysed and I have difficulty chewing or opening my mouth.
>
> (Eve)

Eating is a sin. When it is indulged in both the internal judge of the anorexic will, and the external judge of others' opinion punish it with guilt and shame. The anorexic woman feels caught out, her hidden insatiability revealed. The 'bloated' stomach is symbolic of 'fat': the sign of insatiability.

Wellbourne and Purgold argue that 'fat' for anorexic women equals 'moral decay'; being fat means being 'lazy, greedy, selfish, sloppy, stupid, unattractive, uncaring, untidy and disgusting'

(Wellbourne and Purgold, 1984: 4). I asked the women how they would feel if they were very fat:

> I often imagine being very fat and I would have to hide away in bed for protection. This would be the only way I could hide my body away from people again. I would not be able to cope.
>
> (Eve)

> Awful, I would hide myself from the world.
>
> (Celia)

> It would be absolutely awful. People would always be looking at me. I feel as though I would get in everybody's way. I feel as though my bust would stick out too much.
>
> (Annette)

Similar feelings emerge at the prospect of reaching the weight deemed medically correct for their height:

> I would be full of self-loathing. I would be depressed. I wouldn't be able to face people for fear of their reactions. I would just hide away, disgusted with myself for being so fat.
>
> (Frances)

> Couldn't stand it. Would hide away and not let people see.
>
> (Lisa)

Being at the approved weight, or heavier, means, I would argue, that the secrecy and shame of the act of eating extends to cover the whole body; the 'evidence' in both cases – food and fat – must be concealed. The bloated stomach is the representative of fat-as-sign for the controlled anorexic woman:

> I think I dislike having food in my stomach more than having it in my mouth. I'm always worried it will make my stomach rounded and hence feel 'heavy' and bloated after a meal.
>
> (Andrea)

Asked if they wanted to change anything about their bodies, most focused on stomach, hips and thighs: 'I'd like to be thinner all over but in particular I'd like my tummy to be less pronounced. It sticks out' (Carol). Anne wishes she had 'no bulging stomach'. It's here that food is seen to wreak its worst effects:

> I feel heavy, self-conscious, frightened of putting on weight, scared of my stomach being bloated, unhappy that I've suc-

cumbed . . . Once I have eaten them [forbidden foods] I feel dirty and heavy, and fatter than ever – it's as if I can almost feel the fat from them piling itself up on my hips and thighs, etc.

(Barbara)

I have always feared becoming fat, when I was afraid that my body would never stop expanding.

(Una)

Thinness is a physical demonstration of denial; fat is the sign of indulgence: 'To me, control and thinness go together. Being even a little overweight spells excess and indulgence' (Andrea).

The stigmata is always there, however, even if its external sign is absent. Lisa writes that if she were very fat, she would feel 'more honest, but ugly'. And Sheila explains why she 'eats' only coffee and diet drinks:

Terrified of getting even fatter than I am and therefore hating myself even more – feel so bulbous and insecure fat. Slimmer I have confidence and I love feeling 'empty'. Terrified too of other people realizing how fat I *really* am.'

This, then, is the central irony of anorexia – even when the anorexic woman is thin 'outside', she is 'really' fat 'inside'. Every time she eats this awful truth hovers around her, waiting to be revealed.

OBJECT

I have argued that the feminine body is socially created as the object on which the masculine subject acts, and that women act as 'caretakers' rather than owners of their bodies. Further, I suggested that women's alienation from the body-object is a hidden alienation, concealed both by the idea of the body as a 'given' in nature, and by the formal gender-neutrality of the ideology of individualism. The previous chapter explored these issues through sexuality and reproduction; in this section, and in the concluding chapter the transformations of and negotiations with the object-body which anorexic women make are explored.

A further aim of this section is to point to ways in which anorexic women feel themselves and their bodies to be the objects of the control of others, especially the medical establishment. This experience of powerlessness contrasts sharply with perceptions of anorexic women as domestic tyrants. However, if we accept ana-lyses which see anorexia as itself a strategy of control we can see clearly why attempts to make her eat – benign or otherwise – appear to the anorexic woman as a threat to her control.

I argued above that the alienation of the self from the body, and especially from bodily appetites, is expressed in a usually obscure-ly but occasionally clearly perceived split between the desiring and the desireless body. As we saw in Chapters 2 and 3, anorexia can be described as a two-stage process, in which the symptom is at first consciously set in motion by a strongly perceived self which imposes control on appetite but subsequently 'escapes' the con-scious control of the anorexic woman and 'takes her over'. Anorexia itself, then, comes to be perceived as a force separate from, but internal to the anorexic woman. 'The anorexia' controls her behaviour; she is powerless in the face of her illness and cannot reverse the process which she herself set in motion.

Noelle Caskey, discussing the work of Hilde Bruch, points out that none of Bruch's patients felt that she could control her illness: 'at a certain critical point during the process of weight loss, something at once alien and interior to them took over' (Caskey, 1986: 184). This alien something is described variously: 'a dictator who dominates me', 'a ghost who surrounds me', 'the little man who objects when I eat' (Bruch, 1978: 55–6). The dominant explanation for this process in psychiatry is, of course, biological – biological processes 'take over' and the search for meaning is abandoned (see Bemis, 1978: 611; Slade, 1984). From a sociologi-cal perspective in which 'biological' processes are understood as created in frameworks of social meaning, the anorexic woman's sense of powerlessness clearly must be related to social structure, and in the present context to definitions of the feminine body as an object and of feminine desire as potentially overwhelming the social order. Anorexia, thus, starts from social meaning, and transforms, rather than creates *ex nihilo* an *existing* definition of the feminine body and feminine desire.

Rejecting the 'pathologizing' of anorexia puts meaning back into the anorexic experience. If 'madness' is not abstracted from social structure by describing it as meaningless and incomprehen-sible we must locate it within the same material and ideological structures which shape 'sanity'. The rigid demarcation of 'normal' and 'abnormal' serves political and ideological functions; however, I do not want to follow the critical strand which would describe anorexia as 'the same but more' of what every woman experiences in a patriarchal culture.

I would argue that the anorexic experience does not simply intensify the conflicts between desire and control, dependence and autonomy which characterize women's experience of their bodies and their relationship with food. Rather, anorexic women *transform* the categories through which female experience is created in an attempt to resolve at the level of the body the contradictory demands of individuality and femininity which all women face in a patriarchal and bourgeois culture.

Through an analysis of my own survey material as well as the existing literature, I hope to show that the sense of impersonal control in anorexia centres not on biological take-over but on the desire for food, seen either as a property of the body or as a force in its own right. The controlling force is variously conceptualized as food, appetite, the body or the anorexia itself, but appetite, I would argue, underlies all the categories. Seen as an active force rather than inanimate material, food takes power from the intense desire of which it is the object; the body controls through appetite – it, rather than the self, desires food; and the anorexia controls as *negative* appetite – it is the resistance to desire which gives the illness-as-active-force its power.

The end of anorexia is, then, the complete overturning of the conscious will which began it. The self shrinks from omnipotence to become the object of a force outside of its power. The anorexic woman cannot understand what is happening to her; she is a mystified and powerless object of what she herself set in motion, the victim of her own creation.

In anorexia the controlling force can be conceptualized as wholly magical or supernatural, as Bruch's work shows. In my own survey this was rare, but Andrea did explain how she feels during a binge in a very similar manner: 'I usually feel possessed by some evil spirit who drives me back into the kitchen in search for more.' And Lynne writes that as well as feeling the characteristic tension and anxiety of anorexic eating, she also feels excited: 'because to me food is something magical which has hidden powers of making me feel good sometimes (when I resist) and bad when I eat it.' Here it is the 'magic' of food, rather than her own willpower, which gives satisfaction; but the magic is far from being positive: 'I begin to panic, I want to "shove" the food down before it does me any more harm, I feel very scared just looking at it.'

Caskey, too, comments on food as magically malevolent in anorexia. After pointing out the nutritional expertise common to many anorexic women, she goes on to argue that:

> Once food is inside the anorexic . . . her attitude toward it undergoes a considerable change. It is no longer a matter of numbers or chemical composition; suddenly food is metamorphosed into a dark dragging force that threatens to take over the anorexic, to sink her under suffocating waves of unwanted flesh. To anorexics, food seems to linger ominously in her body; it has a living presence inside them which overpowers them and which they resent.
>
> (Caskey, 1986: 183)

Sometimes the body itself resists the malevolence of food. June speaks of her fear of literally choking when she has food in her mouth:

> I felt as if there was a lump blocking it and not allowing the food in . . . my mouth and throat were dry and choked, I felt I couldn't swallow, I could not taste the food. It seemed to be stuck in my mouth.

Zoe and Lynne also express an unwilled physical resistance to appetite:

> Sometimes it's a terrible effort, my jaw aches, I eat and eat and still the plate is full. Sometimes I cannot eat another mouthful. Sometimes it seems like there are bugs and insects in the food.

> If there is just enough [food] to quell my raging hunger, then that is OK, but if I can feel food actually 'sitting' in my stomach then it feels very uncomfortable, and it plays on my mind.

The resistance to food and its powers is here located in the body rather than being a conscious strategy of the self. There is a struggle going on here different to the conscious war of self and appetite which we saw earlier. Here the struggle is between two forces separate from, but contained in the self – the irresistable force of magically evil food and the immovable object of the resisting body.

One of Hilde Bruch's patients also expresses an understanding of her body functioning independently of conscious control; indeed, for her, it is the *mind* which is 'weak', the body strong:

My body could do anything – it could walk forever and not get tired. My mind was tricky but my body was honest. It knew exactly what to do and I knew exactly what I could do. I felt very powerful on account of my body. My only weakness was my mind.

(Bruch, 1973: 95)

Hunger escapes conscious control as anorexia progresses and becomes ever more an alien force. The questionnaire asked if the women felt that they were in control of their eating, and as we have seen, security of control in anorexia is fundamentally precarious; the slide from you controlling it to it controlling you is remorseless. Here are some replies to the question 'Are you in control of your eating?'

Yes/No! I feel I am in control but also completely controlled by it.

(Alicia)

Occasionally, but usually I feel that food is controlling me . . . If I gave up trying to control my eating, I might as well give up everything else, as food would *totally* dominate my life.

(Lisa)

It felt completely out of control. I was trying to control it, but it felt as if it was controlling me instead.

(Jane)

No – I wish I were – I often feel it's more in control of me.

(Irene)

Appetite comes to be understood, then, as something apart from the real, resisting self:

[I feel] like I'm in a war. Knowing I shouldn't really eat but wanting the food, its comfort, its taste, etc. It's like fighting an addiction. I'm constantly battling with myself, like having one part of my mind arguing with the other all the time.'

(Barbara)

When I eat normally I feel I am not Eleanor but somebody I don't even know myself. I am someone I hate when I eat normally . . . there is something frantic takes over – truly not *me* then.

The self is either controlled by 'anorexia' or through the split between 'hungry self' and 'real self':

> I feel totally at the mercy of anorexia, like a cancer which has grown in me, and at times seems to be winning.
>
> (Lynne)

> Bulimia seems to me an almost logical counterpart to anorexia. It is in control, not you, as in fact anorexia was, and is, an extreme.
>
> (Norma)

> I never feel in any danger of bingeing, and I adhere rigidly to my restricted eating pattern. But this 'control' is an illusion, because in fact my 'willpower' only operates in a negative and masochistic way, and I feel powerless to reverse it. I'm 'programmed'.
>
> (Polly)

> I don't care if I kill myself endeavouring to maintain the weight 'I' choose.
>
> (Annette)

And Sophie explains the process as a split between her 'rational mind' and the part that wants to be very thin.

Wellbourne and Purgold quote 'Della':

> Food assumes a major role in one's life, it dominates all activities. Food and control encircle the self and the self struggles helpless under its command. Knowledge of the self is confused. You do not know if *you* are this strictly imposed control, or if *it* is dominating *you*. You do not know who you are or what. You act, but you don't know if it is you acting or the control . . . Your true status and identity are lost.
>
> (Wellbourne and Purgold, 1984: 18)

For 'Della' the struggle is between 'the rational, intellectual mind' which knows that bodies *need* food and the 'irrational, emotional will' which starves the body:

> the self is battered in the conflict of wills. Is it my self that blindly shouts 'no' to any offer of food that is not yoghurt, banana, apple or muesli? Or is it my self that struggles to assert itself and fails?
>
> (ibid.: 24–5)

Finally, the appetite-as-oppressor can be seen as lodged in the body, which is wholly distinct from and struggling with the self:

> My body craves for food.
>
> (Tracy)

> At adolescence, I was very conscious of my body, over which I felt I was losing control. I enjoyed the feeling of control which vomiting gave me . . . [now] I'm not really aware of it belonging to *me*. I don't think about my body and it doesn't seen to belong to me.
>
> (Alicia)

Zoe talks of her experience as an infant as though speaking about an inanimate object:

> My mother was very controlling, terrified of 'spoiling' the baby, she fed it by the clock and then when she *did* feed it still tried to force it to take more than it wanted.'

The struggle with the appetitive body can be physical as well as psychic (see e.g. Wellbourne and Purgold, 1984: 71–5). Twelve of the women who filled in the questionnaire had tried to hurt or damage the bodies which tormented them:

> For a period of a few months, about twelve years ago, I scratched my face consistently with a needle.
>
> (Polly)

> When I was ill I used to scratch and cut myself. I used to bang and hit my head against a wall. I would let myself get really cold and not bother to put on warm clothes, and would generally neglect myself.'
>
> (Jane)

> I often hit myself hard in the places where I would like to lose weight causing myself to receive large, conspicuous bruises.
>
> (Fiona)

> Stubbed out cigarette ends on my wrist, when I was fat.
>
> (Celia)

Annette used to cut 'tiny pieces' out of her arms at 16, and also ate 'Weed killer. Rat poison. Lead. Mercury', arguing that 'all of these are supposed to ruin your stomach but I don't think I could have taken enough'.

Powerlessness

I would argue that in anorexia the concepts of feminine desire as dangerously threatening patriarchal order and the masculine self and of femininity as self-discipline are translated from sexuality to eating, and from an inter- to an intra-gender process. The struggle between 'male' rationality and 'female' sensuality is played out in the single unit of the anorexic body through the radical splitting of appetite from the conscious control of the self. The anorexic woman then becomes the object of the appetite she set out to eliminate.

When the anorexic woman encounters the medical establishment her carefully created and maintained control is taken away from her and she, her body and her eating become the objects of 'real' external forces in the final irony of anorexia. I am reminded here of Elaine Showalter's comments on the treatment of female 'hysterics' in the nineteenth century, where she argues that the 'benign, protective and custodial' Victorian asylum re-created within its wall the restrictive lives its women patients endured in society (Showalter, 1981: 321).

Similarly, the social powerlessness and lack of control of her own life which leads a woman into anorexia is recreated in medical treatment of anorexia, which, as G.F.M. Russell points out, is rarely specific but is best understood as 'a general management' (Russell, 1977: 280). One such general management regime is described by Julie Dexter, a student nurse, as involving bed-rest, close supervision of meals and drug treatment to suppress 'hyperactivity' (Dexter, 1980: 327). Some psychiatrists do recognize the power struggle between doctor and anorexic patient, but the justification of the risk of death allows even the most perceptive to take her control away from the anorexic woman (see e.g. Wellbourne and Purgold, 1984: 24).[4]

Russell recognizes that compulsory admission has its drawbacks, retarding the development of trust between patient and staff; he recommends that women be 'persuaded' to come into hospital voluntarily. Once 'trust' has been established, the patient is encouraged to hand over control of her eating to staff voluntarily, but in any case, confined to the ward, and with nurses present at meals, discarding food is difficult (Russell, 1977). Bhanji argues that there should be 'no undue emphasis on restrictions and supervision', but rather weight gain plus 'elucidation' or 'correction' of 'the pathological attitudes underlying the illness' (Bhanji, 1980: 324).

Restriction and supervision is, however, precisely what hospitalization means for anorexic women:[5]

> Each time I was admitted to hospital, I was weighed, put on bed rest, I had my belongings taken away from me and told I would be rewarded if I put on weight to target weight . . . as soon as I was discharged I immediately got back down to the weight I was before I went into hospital because I was so frightened of how I felt and looked at their target weight.
>
> (Eve)

> When I reached 5 stone 4 lb, my GP decided I should be hospitalized. Words just cannot convey my bitterness over what happened there . . . The only 'question' they seemed to consider was whether what I was doing was 'deliberate' or not. They forced food down me, telling me how wicked I had been for vomiting. They told me I could leave when I reached 6½ stone. So, I behaved like an angel, soon reached 6½ stone, and was allowed to leave – but I'd been eating everything I could lay my hands on in order to leave – the nurse said excitedly 'Look at your chart – your weight's going up and up – soon it will hit the roof!' This *petrified* me. Of course, the only reason I wanted to leave was so that I could lose all this unwanted weight – and yet I felt *so* guilty, so out of control, so confused.
>
> (Una)

> I was a voluntary patient until I was sectioned, because I would not eat meat and wanted home . . . The more I ate and gained weight, I was allowed special privileges, e.g., getting a bath, hair washed, visitors, up to watch TV, etc . . . It was dreadful. I was fattened up to 8 stone, then released, when they thought I had recovered after I had co-operated, and said what they wanted to hear.
>
> (June)

> Loss of privileges, e.g. no clothes, no baths, no visitors unless I ate. Force feeding by nursing staff – very forcefully and aggressively. Insulin injections. The worst treatment of all was ECT. My psychiatrist knew how much I hated this and so if I did not eat, and continued to lose weight I was threatened with further ECT

[electroconvulsive therapy] . . . I only gained weight as I knew that would be the only way I would get out of hospital.

(Paula)

The end of anorexia is objectification: either appetite or the symptom itself come to control the anorexic woman as a force simultaneously internal and alien. She is responsible for it, but cannot control it: she is its object, powerless to change course. The end of anorexia is precisely the reverse of its original aim to transcend feminine appetite and eliminate its threat to the 'self'. The anorexic woman intends to be a fully individual subject, acting on her environment through the vehicle of the needless and inviolate anorexic body. Instead, the anorexic body remains a mirage which she continually sees in front of her but never reaches. In the end, her individual transformation of the social meanings of the feminine body is no such thing: the object-status of femininity is reasserted. It returns, with a vengeance.

Chapter 8

Conclusion
The anorexic body

I would describe myself as being kind of surrounded with glass
– a kind of *noli me tangere* kind of thing . . . I was painfully turned
in on myself and didn't want human contact, whether it was
touching or whether it was emotional, I just didn't want any
kind of human contact.

(Linda)

M B-L: 'Now *be the food* and tell your body what you are doing
and why.'
Anne: 'I'm your food and I'm going into you now – stuffing you
– making you disgusting – fat. I'm your shame and I'm making
you untouchable. No one will ever touch you now. That's what
you want – that no one will touch you.'
She looked up in surprise.

(quoted in Boskind-Lodahl, 1976: 350)

Anorexia is 'a structure of facades constructed to hide a central
hole of non-being'.

(quoted in Wellbourne and Purgold, 1984: 72)

I know that it [anorexia] is always there to be used as a last resort
and a final act of defiance against the too-closely-impinging
world which may threaten to engulf or annihilate me.

(Macleod, 1981: 160)

In the war against my own body, fatness was not the only or even
the most important enemy . . . I began to get off on not eating,
to enjoy starvation as an end in itself . . . 'I' was the mystical,
starving self, in battle against the base instincts. I would refrain
not just from eating but even from drinking water. Calories
were only the enemy's foot soldiers; the enemy I was fighting

against was my body, my instincts, my desires. And I almost won.

(Valverde, 1985: 33)

Anorexia transforms the social meanings of the body. It works with two opposing body-concepts: the 'individual' (masculine) body as complete in itself, the owned instrument of the individual self or subject, used to act on an environment external to the self and the body; and the feminine body as alienated, incomplete and acted on, a passive/receptive object which, paradoxically, has a simultaneously voracious potential to overwhelm. The individual (masculine) body is 'an active, working thing'; the feminine body is 'a passive vehicle intended to provide gratification', which exists in order to be used, to be consumed (Macleod, 1981: 166; 165–6). Anorexia aims at an individualized transformation of the degraded feminine body in the construction of an anorexic body which is owned, inviolate and needless. The anorexic body, as a personally owned object, is intended to be the body of an active subject; the anorexic symptom intends the transformation of the feminine body-object from its status as the environment on which the masculine subject acts. Its success in achieving this intention is, as we have seen, rare, precarious and temporary: both bodily integrity and bodily instrumentality prove to be ellusive. Desire, however, as Diamond points out, goes beyond the possible (Diamond, 1985: 59).

Anorexia begins as an attempt to control the feminine body in which voracious feminine appetites are lodged. The feminine body, sexually, is the object of the action of others; in eating, however, feminine appetite is, it is thought, under personal control. Desire for women means responsiveness – taking in. The anorexic body, thus, takes in nothing; nothing invades what Wellbourne and Purgold call 'the anorexic fortress' (Wellbourne and Purgold, 1984: 56). The ritualized eating pattern shuts out progressively more and more food; the avoidance of physical contact creates empty space around the anorexic body. It becomes, in Caskey's term, 'a protected zone' (Caskey, 1986: 184), in Douglas's, an 'impermeable . . . container' (Douglas, 1966: 158), in Sheila Macleod's 'cold, untouched and untouchable' (Macleod, 1981: 118).

The anorexic body is empty inside, and emptiness means being clean. It is not contaminated by external things, but is pure. 'Safe' food, food as fuel, is originally distinguished from food as pleasure; in the logic of denial the distinction, as we have seen, collapses and all food is seen as contamination. Food, as Macleod argues, acts in anorexia as a metaphor for 'all foreign substances': 'I remember feeling swollen and polluted after consuming what, to others, would have been a negligible amount of food' (ibid.: 116; 70).

Desire, for women, is constructed as responsive: it means opening up to allow intrusion. Desire, for the ostensibly gender-less individual, is constructed as a move outwards to satisfy internal needs; the body remains whole as it moves out into the world. Feminine desire entails the inclusion of the alien, and expresses the status of women as acted-on environment rather than active subject. The central criterion of the subject is his ability to satisfy his desires through his action on the separate world of objects; he invades and manipulates that environment, it does not invade him. Invasion entails loss of subjecthood; if you are acted on, you are an object, not a subject. Objectification equals the annihilation of the self.

In anorexia the experience of feminine bodily openness is centred on the mouth. Not eating forms a barrier between the anorexic self and the threatening world against which the open feminine body has no defences. Not eating deconstructs feminine responsiveness; it protects against the invasion which threatens to annihilate the self. The anorexic body is a 'fortress' ; it is a 'shell' (Lawrence, 1984a: 22); it contains and protects the self in a way the feminine body can never do.

Desire, for women, is constructed as voracious; feminine desire threatens patriarchal order, it threatens to encompass the (masculine) subject, it threatens chaos. The masculine subject depends for its existence on the construction of the feminine object as an arena for action. Masculine penetration completes the incomplete feminine; feminine incompletion, however, threatens to engulf the intruder. When women threaten to become active subjects, the patriarchal definition of personhood is undermined. Anorexic women are engaged in the project of integrating the individualized/masculine self into the anorexic body, which is feminine; voracious feminine appetites threaten the self and must be eliminated. Feminine desire threatens an end to the dualism of subject and object; feminine appetite is chaotic. 'Fat' is the external sign of voracious appetite; it intrudes into masculine space.

Food is external but appetite, the desire for food, is internal.

Food in anorexia is appetite made concrete. Starvation, then, has two meanings; it intends the elimination of appetite as well as the end of intrusion: 'I dream of the perfect day when I have no appetite, no thought, no desire, or temptation for food or to eat' (quoted in Abraham and Llewellyn-Jones, 1984: 37).

Anorexic emptiness has two meanings. Not eating means nothing is taken in; not wanting to eat means that the desire to take in is eliminated too. The elimination of appetite, then, closes and completes the open and incomplete feminine body around an empty, pure and static inner space. It cannot be acted on; it offers no way in; it is no longer open to the invasion of others. Neither does it threaten to engulf the self. Its elimination allows the 'real' self to appear:

> The clearer the outline of my skeleton became, the more I felt my true self to be emerging, like a nude statue being gradually hewn from some amorphous block of stone.
>
> (Macleod, 1981: 79–80)

Anorexic transformation, however, is an individual transformation of social meaning; what the anorexic woman struggles to contain is not her own appetite but feminine desire. The individual woman cannot negate a social meaning; in the end it comes to control her, either as appetite or as denial. The core process of anorexia is denial; since the anorexic woman is trying to eliminate as an individual a social creation, she can never in her single body deny enough or be thin enough to contain its threat. This, then, is the 'moral spiral' (Turner, 1984) of anorexia. She continues to elaborate her rituals of denial in a never ending spiral, and never finally and securely reaches the place where, with personal control of her body as an object, she could begin to act as a subject.

The empty and inviolate anorexic body is the ideal end of the anorexic process; few anorexic women ever achieve it. Existence in the anorexic body is grasped momentarily; it continually slips away. The road to the anorexic body has two detours, both dead ends. In the first, appetite controls the anorexic woman directly. Characterized as non-human, it overwhelms the self in binges and fantasies of binges; anorexia here is the continual attempt to impose denial on an appetite perceived as unstoppable, as, in Caskey's term, a force 'at once alien and interior' (Caskey, 1986: 184). Here, 'fat' in general and the 'bloated' stomach in particular are signs of the failure of anorexic discipline in the face of an appetite which is alien to the anorexic woman but which is nevertheless her responsibility. Wellbourne and Purgold quote 'Petra':

> It's the feeling of how dirty you are inside that makes you feel it must show outside, which may account for the fact I'm not happy unless I am slim enough to see my bones, 'the real me'.
>
> (quoted in Wellbourne and Purgold, 1984: 110)

Flesh, then, is appetite made concrete: it is 'something swollen, polluted, dirty' (Macleod, 1981: 69). Flesh is the feminine body; the skeleton contains the anorexic self. Anorexia aims at the transcendence of appetite; its most common outcome is a never-ending struggle with appetite and its sign, flesh.

In the second anorexic detour, appetite controls indirectly. The symptom itself, not-eating, negative appetite, comes to control the anorexic woman; she feels herself powerless to end a process she herself began. Sheila Macleod writes: 'I didn't know what I was doing: I just felt compelled to do it' (ibid.: 10). And Wellbourne and Purgold's 'Della' explains:

> You do not know if *you* are this strictly imposed control, or if it is dominating *you*. You do not know who you are or what. You act, but you don't know if it is you acting or the control. Both come from within and mingle together in an inseparable fusion.
>
> (quoted in Wellbourne and Purgold, 1984: 18)

The denial which she participates in is itself, of course, a social construction. Feminine self-discipline is the self-policing of feminine desire, and is one element in the social control of feminine desire. Like appetite, then, denial is a social force; what the anorexic woman struggles with is not her own denial but a social control. Her original resistance to her incorporation in the degraded feminine body rises up, and with phantom substantiality, controls its creator.

The reality of anorexia, then, entails a re-objectification of the feminine body, which becomes the object either of interior-but-alien appetite or interior-but-alien anorexia.[1] The anorexic woman thinks, accepting the definition of the body as individually owned, that her body is the one thing she can control. The object status of the feminine body is, however, ultimately, inescapable. The subject in bourgeois patriarchal culture is a consuming subject; acting to satisfy its desires, in its own self-interest, is what defines it; it wants, therefore it is. Women, as the environment of the masculine subject, have, ultimately, no wholly separate environment on which to act, since they are part of the world of objects in opposition to which the individualized subject is constructed: women desire to be possessed as objects. Possessive desire as subjects is constructed, for women, as non-willed, non-human. It is not controlled by a true subject: it will overwhelm, rather than express, the self.

There is, then, a fundamental internal limit to the gender-neutral individuality at which anorexia aims. Women cannot desire as subjects; women are objects; women are bodies. In anorexia women are the objects of a socially constructed feminine voraciousness; or they are the objects of the social control of feminine voraciousness. They cannot be wholly subjects. Desire, active and fulfillable, defines the self; anorexia aims to eliminate desire, and in so doing eliminates the self. The desireless anorexic body ultimately contains nothing: 'towards the climax of the disease, there was very little of me left, in more than the physiological sense' (Macleod, 1981: 108).

Anorexia is an attempt to resolve at the level of the individual body the irreconcilability of individuality and femininity in a bourgeois patriarchal culture. It works indirectly, because it works with largely hidden social meanings, meanings which feminism has begun to unearth from bourgeois patriarchal ideology.

Kim Chernin, as we have seen, argues that patriarchal culture has opened its doors to women in response to feminist pressure (Chernin, 1986). In Chapter 3 I criticized this claim, arguing that it owes more to bourgeois ideology than to actual practice. The 'equal opportunities' culture suggests that women can now compete, as individuals, for wealth, status and power. The ideology of bourgeois individualism conceals the structural constraints on individual achievement. In its gender-neutral incarnation, the masking of the reality of class relations extends to mask the reality of gender relations: we live in the era of 'post-feminism'.

Post-feminist theorists claim that the individualistic pursuit of self-interest is now as open to women as it is to men. White middle-class women, because of their specific location in gender, class and ethnic relations, are the special objects of post-feminist ideology, since a relatively privileged class position combines with the benefits of being white in a racist social order to allow them increased access to career success and public position. But the closer they get, the more directly the inherent limits of 'gender-neutral' individualism are experienced.

White middle-class women who reach adulthood in the equal opportunities culture must personally reconcile this contradiction; they must create a sense of self in which individuality and femininity can coexist. Anorexia is one attempt at such a reconciliation. Feminism brings the contradiction into the light of political discourse partially and fitfully; feminist analyses give some women the opportunity to directly and collectively grapple with the continuing realities of patriarchal oppression. But feminism's alternative social analysis exists in a social order which bourgeois patriarchal ideology already structures and makes sense of. Feminist explanations and resistances are continually undercut, and a bourgeois and patriarchal individualism reasserted.

We can see an example of this in Wellbourne and Purgold's proto-feminist analysis of anorexia. Wellbourne and Purgold argue that:

> the pressures and demands of . . .'society' on young women are more confused and internally self-contradictory than the equivalent pressures and demands on young men . . . adult autonomy is acquired in different ways and to different degrees by boys and by girls and . . . the acquisition of autonomy by girls gets a more mixed reception from adult observers.
>
> (Wellbourne and Purgold, 1984: 114, 117)

This situation, however, is *not* an outcome of a patriarchal social order for Wellbourne and Purgold. They argue that such pressures arise from 'the social imperatives of yesteryear' affecting 'parental policy' (ibid.: 115). It is an outdated and faulty upbringing, then, rather than the social control of women, which leads the 'pre-anorexic' girl to feel that she has no 'personal rights' (ibid.: 112). Therapeutic intervention will give the anorexic women what 'most of us who are not anorexic' have; that is, a 'central "core" self' which allows us to regulate and prioritize individual needs and the demands of others (ibid.: 120). It will teach the anorexic woman that autonomy is both possible and acceptable (ibid.:128).

The argument that autonomy and femininity are not reconcilable, then, is presented only to be explained away as outmoded tradition and familial pathology. The dilemma which the anorexic woman feels is not 'real'; it is one which the more competent upbringing that 'most of us' have had resolves naturally as we reach 'maturity' (ibid.: 128). Even in more fully feminist analyses of anorexia, as we saw in Chapter 3, individual therapy which will 're-nurture' women into true individuality is suggested as a solution to the anorexic dilemma. If, however, we understand anorexia as an individualized 'solution' to a cultural contradiction we can see more clearly that its ultimate strategic failure is explained by its very individualization. My contention in this book is that we cannot fully understand the anorexic symptom without an analysis of the structures of social meaning and social practices in bourgeois patriarchal culture; only a collective feminist engagement with those meanings and practices *as social* can transform the subjection of women which leads to anorexia.

Notes

INTRODUCTION

1 Analyses of anorexia which focus on the social situation of women are criticized for their inability to explain why *all* middle-class teenage girls do not become anorexic. This critique rests on determinist assumptions, suggesting that social position determines a single course of action. Rather than being the one inescapable response to patriarchal social structure, anorexia, I would argue, is one of a range of 'solutions' to the irreconcilability of individuality and femininity. I am not concerned to explain why 'woman A' becomes anorexic while 'woman B' becomes a feminist; rather, my concern is to establish the political meaning of anorexia as one engagement with the dilemmas of patriarchy.

2 I am not suggesting that de Beauvoir takes a social constructionist view of the body, but that her work can be used in the development of such a perspective; see Evans, 1983.

3 For a discussion of different uses of the concept of difference in sociology see Barrett, 1987. Here I am using the concept in Barrett's second sense: difference as constructed through opposition.

4 There are a number of autobiographical accounts of anorexia – see Havekamp, 1978; Macleod, 1981; O'Neill, 1982; Roche, 1984; Wilkinson, 1984; Garfield, 1986; Waugh, 1988.

1 ANOREXIA NERVOSA: THE HISTORY OF THE CONCEPT

1 See also Baglivi, 1723 and Mexio, 1613.

2 Medieval constructions of the body are discussed in Chapter 5.

2   THE ENIGMA VARIATIONS: PSYCHIATRIC EXPLANATIONS OF ANOREXIA

1   See, for example, Mora on 'the basic consistency of human needs and ways of solving problems' (quoted in Penfold and Walker, 1983: 10).
2   'Modern' is undefined here, but from its context we can assume Crisp is referring to the 1960s onwards (1967: 715).
3   It is not helpful, I would argue, to pursue this point further since, as a sociologist, I am not competent in this area. While I cannot disprove organic theories of causation in anorexia on biological grounds, in Part III I hope to provide both an adequate critique of sociobiology and a more illuminating sociological explanation of anorexia.

3   WOMEN'S OPPRESSION: FEMINIST EXPLANATIONS OF ANOREXIA

1   To take only one example, feminist sociologists have detailed the split into private/female and public/male worlds during the transition from feudalism to capitalism, pointing out that that dichotomy is itself historical rather than universal (see e.g. Rowbotham, 1977; Hamilton, 1978).
2   Lawrence argues that the middle-class bias in anorexia is in fact educational; it is this specific feature of middle-class experience rather than class position *per se* which fosters anorexia (Lawrence, 1984b: 201–2).
3   For discussion on the extent to which this is the case see e.g. Segal, 1987; Dworkin, 1988.

5   THE SOCIOLOGY OF THE BODY

1   Using Turner's framework does not, of course, force one to reach his conclusions, and I am especially critical of his arguments on patriarchy (ibid.: 120–56) and their conclusion that differentiation of bodies by gender is becoming increasingly irrelevant (ibid.: 29).
2   For an alternative view see Degler, 1973; as Degler correctly points out, social prohibitions do not necessarily describe actual behaviour, and we should not assume an absence of resistance. Here, however, it is the ideology which interests me.

6   THE FEMININE BODY

1   Millett sees 'human consciousness' (1977: 63) as the basis of patriarchy and thus, I would argue, too readily dismisses patriarchal institutions and material practices, slipping into idealism (see Kaplan, 1986). In discussing patriarchal ideology, however, her work was pioneering and remains extremely useful.
2   Griffin points out that 'chastity' is not the only criterion for distin-

guishing 'rapable' and 'unrapable' women; black women tend to be categorized as 'unrapable' regardless, due to their racist categorization as 'impure' (Griffin, 1971: 5–6).

3   Elizabeth Arden, 'Cabriole', quoted in Williamson (1985: 27).

4   Quotations in this section are taken from skincare adverts in a random selection of women's magazines, and are identified by product.

5   Tickner (1976) and Henley (1977) explore the restriction of the female body in, respectively, clothing and movement.

7   THE ANOREXIC SYMPTOM

1   The other main explanation was that the anorexia was her way of coping with 'deeper' difficulties and problems, usually seen as familial; while not a direct control explanation the two are obviously related.

2   For a discussion of recovery see Hsu, 1980.

3   Crisp points out that in his experience carbohydrates are cut out first, and then progressively more and more types of food (Crisp, 1970a: 467).

4   For differing views on the risk of death in anorexia, see Hsu, 1980: 1042; Norton, 1983: 318; Wellbourne and Purgold, 1984: 9.

5   Though most of the women in the survey were to say the least critical of the treatment they received, as we saw in Chapter 4, if the woman can bring herself to hand over control of her eating willingly it can be quite a relief: 'I was desperate to come out of the disorder. I was relieved that the doctor told me to indulge...' (Norma). And psychotherapy in general was significantly more highly valued than treatment which concentrated mainly on weight gain.

8   CONCLUSION: THE ANOREXIC BODY

1   My argument here is indebted to Gabel's incisive analysis of schizophrenia, in which, following Marx, he suggests that the position of the human subject as the object of capitalist social relations is transformed and re-experienced in schizophrenic 'withdrawal' (Gabel, 1975: see, especially, p. 146; Marx, 1953: 77).

Bibliography

Abraham, S. and Llewellyn-Jones, D. (1984) *Eating Disorders: The Facts*, Oxford University Press.

Adams, P. (1986) 'Versions of the body', *m/f*, 11/12.

Alexander, S. and Taylor, B. (1979) 'In defence of "patriarchy"', *New Statesman*, 28 Dec.

Anderson, A. E. (1977) 'Atypical anorexia nervosa', in R. A. Vigersky (ed.) *Anorexia Nervosa*, Raven Press.

Ardener, S. (ed.) (1978) *Defining Females: The Nature of Women in Society*, London, Croom Helm.

Arditti, R., Duelli Klein, R. and Minden, S. (eds) (1984) *Test-tube Women: What Future for Motherhood?*, London, Pandora.

Ariès, P. (1973) *Centuries of Childhood*, Harmondsworth, Penguin.

Arieti, S. (1947) 'The two aspects of schizophrenia', *Psychiatric Quarterly*, 31.

Arnold, K. (1978) 'The whore in Peru', in S. Lipschitz (ed.) *Tearing the Veil: Essays on Femininity*, London, Routledge & Kegan Paul.

Atkinson, P. (1983) 'Eating virtue', in A. Murcott (ed.) *The Sociology of Food and Eating*, Aldershot, Gower.

Baglivi, G. (1723) *The Practice of Physick*, London.

Bakhtin, M. (1968) *Rabelais and His World*, Cambridge, MA, MIT Press.

Bardwick, J. M. and Douvan, E. (1971) 'Ambivalence: the socialisation of women', in V. Gornick and B. K. Moran (eds) *Women in Sexist Society*, New York, Basic Books.

Barker-Benfield, G. J. (1973) 'The spermatic economy: a 19th-century view of sexuality', in M. Gordon (ed.) *The American Family in Social Historical Perspective*, New York, St Martin's Press.

Barker-Benfield, G. J. (1976) *The Horrors of the Half-known Life: Male Attitudes toward Women and Sexuality in 19th-century America*, New York, Harper & Rowe.

Barrett, M. (1980) *Women's Oppression Today*, London, Verso/NLB.

Barrett, M. (1987) 'The concept of difference', *Feminist Review*, 26.

Beechey, V. (1979) 'On patriarchy', *Feminist Review*, 3.

Bell, R. M. (1985) *Holy Anorexia*, Chicago, University of Chicago Press.

Bemis, K. M. (1978) 'Current approaches to the etiology and treatment of anorexia nervosa', *Psychological Bulletin*, 85 (3).

Bhanji, S. (1980) 'Anorexia nervosa: two schools of thought', *Nursing Times*, 78 (8).

Birke, L. and Silvertown, J. (eds) (1984) *More than the Parts: Biology and Politics*, London, Pluto.

Black, M. and Coward, R. (1981) 'Man-made language: linguistic, social and sexual relations', *Screen Education*, 39.

Bland, L. (1981) 'The domain of the sexual: a response', *Screen Education*, 39.

Bolton, B. M. (1978) 'Vitae matrum: a further aspect of the frauenfrage', in D. Baker (ed.) *Medieval Women*, Oxford, Blackwell.

Booth, W. C. (1982) 'Freedom of interpretation: Bakhtin and the challenge of feminist criticism', *Critical Inquiry*, 9.

Boskind-Lodahl, M. (1976) 'Cinderella's step-sisters: a feminist perspective on anorexia nervosa and bulimia', *Signs: a Journal of Women in Culture and Society*, 2 (2).

Box, S. (1983) *Power, Crime and Mystification*, London, Tavistock.

British Sociological Association Equality of the Sexes Committee (1987) 'Proceedings of BSA Equality of the Sexes Committee workshop on women and research', November.

Brooke, C. L. N. (1978) 'Both small and great beasts: an introductory study', in D. Baker (ed.) *Medieval Women*, Oxford, Blackwell.

Brooke, R. and Brooke, C. L. N. (1978) 'St Clare', in D. Baker (ed.) *Medieval Women*, Oxford, Blackwell.

Broverman, I. *et al.* (1970) 'Sex-role stereotypes and clinical judgement', *The Journal of Clinical and Consulting Psychiatry*, 34.

Broverman, I. *et al.* (1972) 'Sex-role stereotypes: a reappraisal', *Journal of Social Issues*, 28.

Brown, B. and Adams, P. (1979) 'The feminine body and feminist politics', *m/f*, 3.

Brownmiller, S. (1978) *Against Our Will: Men, Women and Rape*, Harmondsworth, Penguin.

Bruch, H. (1961) 'Conceptual confusion in eating disorders', *Journal of Nervous and Mental Diseases*, 133.

Bruch, H. (1969) 'Hunger and instinct', *Journal of Nervous and Mental Disease*, 149 (2).

Bruch, H. (1970) 'Changing approaches to anorexia nervosa', *International Psychiatric Clinics*, 7 (1).

Bruch, H. (1971) 'Family transactions in eating disorders', *Comprehensive Psychiatry*, 12 (3).

Bruch, H. (1974) *Eating Disorders: Obesity, Anorexia Nervosa and the Person Within*, London, Routledge & Kegan Paul.

Bruch, H. (1975) 'Obesity and anorexia nervosa: psychosocial aspects', *Australian and New Zealand Journal of Psychiatry*, 9.

Bruch, H. (1977) 'Psychological antecedents of anorexia nervosa', in R. A. Vigersky (ed.) *Anorexia Nervosa*, Raven Press.

Bruch, H. (1978) *The Golden Cage: The Enigma of Anorexia*, Wells, Open Books.

Bruch, H. (1980) 'Preconditions for the development of anorexia nervosa', *American Journal of Psychoanalysis*, 40 (2).

Bruch, H. (1982) 'Anorexia nervosa: therapy and theory', *American Journal of Psychiatry*, 139 (12).

Brunsdon, C. (1978) '"It is well known that by nature women are inclined to be rather personal"', in Women's Studies Group, CCCS (eds) *Women Take Issue*, London, Hutchinson.

BSSRS Sociobiology Group (1984) 'Human sociobiology', in L. Birke and J. Silvertown (eds) *More than the Parts: Biology and Politics*, London, Pluto.

Burniston, S., Mort, F. and Weedon, C. (1978) 'Psychoanalysis and the cultural acquisition of sexuality and subjectivity', in Women's Studies Group, CCCS (eds) *Women Take Issue*, London, Hutchinson.

Cameron, D. and Frazer, E. (1987) *The Lust to Kill: a Feminist Investigation of Sexual Murder*, Cambridge, Polity Press.

Caputi, J. (1987) *The Age of Sex Crime*, London, Women's Press.

Caskey, N. (1986) 'Interpreting anorexia nervosa', in S. Suleiman (ed.) *The Female Body in Western Culture: Contemporary Perspectives*, Cambridge, MA, Harvard University Press.

Casper, R. C. *et al.* (1980) 'Bulimia: its incidence and clinical importance in patients with anorexia nervosa', *Archives of General Psychiatry*, 37.

Chambers, G. and Miller, A. (1983) *Investigating Sexual Assault: A Scottish Office Research Study*, HMSO.

Chambers, G. and Miller, A. (1987) *Prosecuting Sexual Assault: A Scottish Office Research Study*, HMSO.

Chapkis, W. (1986) *Beauty Secrets: Women and the Politics of Appearance*, Boston, South End Press.

Chernin, K. (1983) *Womansize: The Tyranny Of Slenderness*, London, Women's Press.

Chernin, K. (1986) *Women, eating and identity*, London, Virago.

Chesler, P. (1974) *Women and Madness*, Allen Lane.

Chiodo, J. and Latimer, K. (1983) 'Vomiting as a learned weight-control technique in bulimia', *Journal of Behavioural Therapy & Experimental Psychology*, 14 (2).

Clark, L. and Lewis, D. (1977) *Rape: The Price of Coercive Sexuality*, Women's Press (Canada).

Cooper, J. (1977) *Harriet*, London, Corgi.

Corea, G. (1985) *The Mother-machine: Reproductive Technologies from Artificial Insemination to Artificial Wombs*, New York, Harper & Rowe.

Cousins, M. and Hussain, A. (1984) *Michel Foucault*, London, Macmillan.

Coward, R. (1982) 'Sexual violence and sexuality', *Feminist Review*, 11.

Coward, R. (1984) *Female Desire*, London, Paladin.

Cowie, E. and Lees, S. (1981) 'Slags or drags?', *Feminist Review*, 9.

Crisp, A. H. (1967) 'Anorexia nervosa', *Hospital Medicine*, 1.

Crisp, A. H. (1968) 'Primary anorexia nervosa', *Gut*, 9.

Crisp, A. H. (1970a) 'Premorbid factors in adult disorders of weight, with particular reference to primary anorexia nervosa (weight phobia). A literature review.', *Journal of Psychosomatic Research*, 14.

Crisp, A. H. (1970b) 'Anorexia nervosa: "feeding disorder", "nervous malnutrition" or "weight phobia"?', *World Review of Nutrition and Dietetics*, 12.

Crisp, A. H. (1974) 'Primary anorexia nervosa or adolescent weight phobia', *The Practitioner*, 212.

Crisp, A. H. (1977) 'Some psychobiological aspects of adolescent growth and their relevance for the fat/thin syndrome (anorexia nervosa)', *International Journal of Obesity*, 1.

Crisp, A. H. (1979) 'Anorexia nervosa: a disease of our time. (The need to make provision for it)', *Health and Hygiene*, 2 (3).

Crisp, A. H. (1980) *Anorexia Nervosa: Let Me Be*, Academic Press.

Crisp, A. H. (1981–2) 'Anorexia nervosa at normal body weight: The abnormal normal weight control syndrome', *International Journal of Psychiatry in Medicine*, 11 (3).

Crisp, A. H. (1983a) 'Anorexia nervosa', *British Medical Journal*, 287 (24 Sept.).

Crisp, A. H. (1983b) 'Psychologically crippling condition', *British Medical Journal*, 287, (17 Sept.).

Crisp, A. H. and Bhat, A. V. (1982) '"Personality" and anorexia nervosa: the phobic avoidance stance, its origins and its symptomatology', *Psychotherapy and Psychosomatics*, 38.

Crisp, A. H. and Fransella, F. (1972) 'Conceptual changes during recovery from anorexia nervosa', *British Journal of Medical Psychology*, 45.

Crisp, A. H. and Fransella, F. (1979) 'Comparisons of weight concepts in groups of neurotic, normal and anorexic females', *British Journal of Psychiatry*, 134.

Crisp, A. H. and Hsu, L. K. G. (1980) 'The Crown–Crisp Experiential Index (CCEI) profile in anorexia nervosa', *British Journal of Psychiatry*, 136.

Crisp, A. H., Hsu, L. K. G. and Harding, B. (1980) 'The starving hoarder and the voracious spender: stealing in anorexia nervosa', *Journal of Psychosomatic Research*, 24.

Crisp, A. H. and Kalucy, R. S. (1974) 'Aspects of the perceptual disorder in anorexia nervosa', *British Journal of Medical Psychology*, 47.

Crisp, A. H., Kalucy, R. S., Lacey, J. H. and Harding, B. (1977) 'The long-term prognosis in anorexia nervosa: some factors predictive of outcome', in R. A. Vigersky (ed.) *Anorexia Nervosa*, Raven Press.

Dally, P. and Gomez, J. (1980) *Obesity and Anorexia Nervosa: A Question of Shape*, London, Faber.

Dana, M. and Lawrence, M. (1987) '"Poison is the nourishment that makes one ill": the metaphor of bulimia', in M. Lawrence (ed.) *Fed Up and Hungry: Women, Oppression and Food*, London, Women's Press.

de Beauvoir, S. (1972) *The Second Sex*, Harmondsworth, Penguin.

Degler, C. N. (1973) 'What ought to be and what was: women's sexuality in the nineteenth century', in M. Gordon (ed.) *The American Family in Social-historical Perspective*, New York, St Martin's Press.

Deleuze, G. and Guattari, F. (1977) *Anti-Oedipus: Capitalism and Schizophrenia*, Viking.

Dexter, J. M. (1980) 'Anorexia nervosa: a nursing care study', *Nursing Times*, 78 (8).

Diamond, N. (1985) 'Thin is the feminist issue', *Feminist Review*, 19.

Dobash, R. E. and Dobash, R. (1980) *Violence Against Wives: A Case Against the Patriarchy*, Wells, Open Books.

Doerner, K. (1981) *Madmen and the Bourgeoisie*, Oxford, Blackwell.

Douglas, M. (1966) *Purity and Danger: An Analysis of the Concepts of Pollution and Taboo*, London, Routledge & Kegan Paul.

Douglas, M. (1970) *Natural Symbols*, Barrie & Rockliffe: the Cresset Press.

Douglas, M. (1971) 'Do dogs laugh? A cross-cultural approach to body symbolism', *Journal of Psychosomatic Research*, 15.

Dworkin, A. (1974) *Woman Hating*, Dutton.

Dworkin, A. (1981) *Pornography: Men Possessing Women*, London, Women's Press.

Dworkin, A. (1982) 'The rape atrocity and the boy next door', in A. Dworkin (ed.) *Our Blood: Prophecies and Discources on Sexual Politics*, London, Women's Press.

Dworkin, A. (1987) *Intercourse*, Secker & Warburg.

Dworkin, A. (1988) 'Dangerous and deadly', *Trouble and Strife*, 14.

ERCC (Edinburgh Rape Crisis Centre) (1988) 'Legal notes', unpublished.

Ehrenreich, B. and English, D. (1973) *Complaints and Disorders: The Sexual Politics of Sickness*, London, Writers & Readers.

Ehrenreich, B. and English, D. (1979) *For Her Own Good: 150 Years of the Experts' Advice to Women*, London, Pluto.

Ellis, R. (1983) 'The way to a man's heart: food in the violent home', in A. Murcott (ed.) *The Sociology of Food and Eating*, Aldershot, Gower.

Ellmann, M. (1979) *Thinking About Women*, London, Virago.

Evans, M. (1983) 'Simone de Beauvoir: dilemmas of a feminist radical', in D. Spender (ed.) *Feminist Theorists*, London, Women's Press.

Ferguson, M. (1983) *Forever Feminine: Women's Magazines and the Cult of Femininity*, London, Heinemann.

Foucault, M. (1965) *Madness and Civilization*, New York, Pantheon Books.

Foucault, M. (1979) *The History of Sexuality, Volume 1: An Introduction*, London, Allen Lane.

Foucault, M. (1980) *Power/Knowledge: Selected Interviews and Other Writings, 1972–1977*, Brighton, Harvester.

Frazer, E. (1988) 'Teenage girls talking about class', *Sociology: The Journal of the British Sociological Association*, 22 (3).

Gabel, J. (1975) *False Consciousness*, Oxford, Blackwell.

Gallagher, J. (1987) 'Eggs, embryos and foetuses: anxiety and the law', in M. Stanworth (ed.) *Reproductive Technologies: Gender, Motherhood and Medicine*, Cambridge, Polity.

Gamarnikow, E. and Purvis, J. (1985) 'Introduction', in E. Gamarnikow et al., *The Public and the Private*, London, Heinemann.

Gamarnikow, E. *et al.*, (1985) *The Public and the Private*, London, Heinemann.

Garfield, R. (1986) *The Life of a Real Girl: An Autobiography of Anorexia and Madness*, London, Sidgwick & Jackson.

Garfinkel, P. E., Moldofsky, H. and Garner, D. M. (1980) 'The heterogeneity of anorexia nervosa: bulimia as a distinct subgroup', *Archives of General Psychiatry*, 37.

Gottlieb, R. (1984) 'Mothering and the reproduction of power: Chodorow, Dinnerstein and social theory', *Socialist Review*, 14 (5).

Grant, C. (1987) 'Give your skin the works', *Woman's World* (July).

Greer, G. (1971) *The Female Eunuch*, London, Granada.

Griffin, S. (1971) 'Rape: the all-American crime', *Ramparts*, 10 (3).

Griffin, S. (1979) *Rape: The Power of Consciousness*, New York, Harper & Rowe.

Gull, W. W. (1868) 'The Address in Medicine delivered before the Annual Meeting of the British Medical Association, at Oxford', *Lancet*, 8 Aug.

Gull, W. W. (1873) 'Report to the Clinical Society', *Medical Times and Gazette*, 8 Nov.

Gull, W. W. (1874) 'Anorexia Nervosa (Apepsia Hysterica, Anorexia Hysterica)', *Transactions of the Clinical Society of London*, 7.

Gurevich, A. J. (1985) *The Categories of Medieval Culture*, London, Routledge & Kegan Paul.

Hall, J. D. (1984) '"The mind that burns in each body": women, rape, and racial violence', in A. Snitow, S. Stansell and S. Thompson (eds) *Desire: The Politics of Sexuality*, London, Virago.

Hall, R. E. (1985) *Ask Any Woman: A London Inquiry Into Rape and Sexual Assault*, Falling Wall Press.

Hamilton, R. (1978) *The Liberation of Women*, London, Allen & Unwin.

Harvie, L. T. S. (1986) 'The myths about rape and their influence on police procedures', unpublished MA dissertation, Strathclyde University.

Havekamp, K. (1978) *Love Comes in Buckets*, London, Marion Boyars.

Haw, C. and Parker, R. (1977) 'Feminist therapists talking', *Spare Rib*, 61.

Henley, N. (1977) *Body Politics: Power, Sex and Nonverbal Communication*, Prentice-Hall.

Hertz, R. (1960) *Death and the Right Hand*, Cohen & West.

Herzlich, C. (1973) *Health and Illness: A Social-psychological Analysis*, Academic Press.

Hirschon, R. (1978) 'Open body/closed space: the transformation of female sexuality', in S. Ardener (ed.) *Defining Females: The Nature of Women in Society*, London, Croom Helm.

Holdsworth, C. J. (1978) 'Christina of Markyate', in D. Baker (ed.) *Medieval Women*, Oxford, Blackwell.

Hollway, W. (1981) '"I just wanted to kill a woman" Why?', *Feminist Review*, 9.

Hsu, L. K. G. (1980) 'Outcome of anorexia nervosa', *Archives of General Psychiatry*, 37.

Hudson, B. (1984) 'Femininity and adolescence', in A. McRobbie and M. Nava (eds) *Gender and Generation*, Macmillan.

Imray, L. and Middleton, A. (1983) 'Public and private: marking the boundaries', in A. Murcott (ed.) *The Sociology of Food and Eating*, Aldershot, Gower.

Kaplan, C. (1986) *Sea Changes: Culture and Feminism*, London, Verso.

Kelly, L. (1987) 'The new defeatism', *Trouble & Strife*, 11.

Kitzinger, C. (1987) *The Social Construction of Lesbianism*, London, Sage.

Klein, M. (1975) *The Psychoanalysis of Children*, London, Hogarth.

Klibansky, R., Saxl, F., and Panofsky, E. (1964) *Saturn and Melancholy: Studies in the History of Natural Philosphy, Religion and Art*, Nelson.

Lasègue, E. (1873) 'On Hysterical Anorexia', *Medical Times and Gazette*, 6 Sept.

Lawrence, M. (1979) 'Anorexia nervosa: the control paradox', *Women's Studies International Quarterly*, 2.

Lawrence, M. (1984a) *The Anorexic Experience*, London, Women's Press.

Lawrence, M. (1984b) 'Education and identity: thoughts on the social origins of anorexia', *Women's Studies International Forum*, 7 (4).

Lawrence, M. (ed.) (1987) *Fed Up and Hungry: Women, Oppression and Food*, London, Women's Press.

Lees, S. (1986) *Losing Out: Sexuality and Adolescent Girls*, London, Hutchinson.

Leyser, H. (1984) *Hermits and the New Monasticism: A Study of Religious Communities in Western Europe, 1000–1150*, London, Macmillan.

Lipschitz, S. (1978) 'The witch and her devils: an exploration of the relationship between femininity and illness', in S. Lipschitz (ed) *Tearing the Veil: Essays on Femininity*, London, Routledge & Kegan Paul.

Lloyd, G. (1984) *The Man of Reason: 'Male' and 'Female' in Western Philosophy*, London, Methuen.

Lourdaux, W. and Verhelst, D. (1976) *The Concept of Heresy in the Middle Ages*, Leuven, Leuven University Press.

LRCC (London Rape Crisis Centre) (1984) *Sexual Violence: The Reality for Women*, London, Women's Press.

Macleod, S. (1981) *The Art of Starvation*, London, Virago.

Marx, K. (1953) *Capital*, Vol. 1, Lawrence & Wishart.

Mauss, M. (1973) (Orig. 1935) 'The techniques of the body', *Economy and Society*, 2 (1).

Mexio, P. (1613) *The Treasurie of Ancient and Modern Times*, Jaggard.

Miller, J. B. (1976) *Towards a New Psychology of Women*, Allen Lane.

Miller, N. K. (1986) 'Rereading as a woman: the body in practice', in S. Suleiman (ed.) *The Female Body in Western Culture: Contemporary Perspectives*, Cambridge, MA, Harvard University Press.

Millett, K. (1977) *Sexual Politics*, London, Virago.

Moore, R. J. (1976) 'Heresy and disease', in W. Lourdaux and D. Verhelst (eds), *The Concept of Heresy in the Middle Ages*, Leuven, Leuven University Press.

Morgan, H. G. (1977) 'Fasting girls and our attitudes to them', *British Medical Journal*, 2.

Morgan, H. G., Purgold, J. and Wellbourne, J. (1983) 'Management and outcome in anorexia nervosa: a standardized prognostic study', *British Journal of Psychiatry*, 143.

Morton, R. (1694) *Pthisiologia: Or, a Treatise of Consumptions*, Sam. Smith and Benj. Walford. University Microfilms International, Ann Arbor, MI, 48106.

Murcott, A. (ed.) (1983a) *The Sociology of Food and Eating*, Aldershot, Gower.

Murcott, A. (1983b) 'Cooking and the cooked: a note on the domestic preparation of meals', in A. Murcott (ed.) *The Sociology of Food and Eating*, Aldershot, Gower.

Murcott, A. (1983c) "'It's a pleasure to cook for him": food, mealtimes and gender in some South Wales households', in A. Murcott (ed.) *The Sociology of Food and Eating*, Aldershot, Gower.

Norton, K. (1983) 'Anorexia nervosa', *Midwife, Health Visitor and Community Nurse*, 19.

Oakley, A. (1974) *The Sociology of Housework*, Robertson.

Oakley, A. (1981) *Subject Women*, Robertson.

Oakley, A. (1987) 'From walking wombs to test-tube babies', in M. Stanworth (ed.) *Reproductive Technologies: Gender, Motherhood and Medicine*, Cambridge, Polity.

O'Neill, C. B. (1982) *Starving for Attention*, Continuum.

Orbach, S. (1978) *Fat is a Feminist Issue*, London, Hamlyn.

Orbach, S. (1986) *Hunger Strike: The Anorectic's Struggle as a Metaphor for Our Age*, London, Faber & Faber.

Orbach, S. and Eichenbaum, L. (1983) *Understanding Women*, Harmondsworth, Penguin.

Palazzoli, M. S. (1967) 'Die Bildung des Korperbewussteins: die Ernahrung des Kindes als Lernprozess', *Psychotherapy and Psychosomatics*, 15.

Palazzoli, M. S. (1969) 'Die Bildung des Korperbewussteins II', *Psychotherapy and Psychosomatics*, 17.

Palazzoli, M. S. (1974) *Self-starvation: From the Intrapsychic to the Transpersonal Approach to Anorexia Nervosa*, Human Context Books.

Palmer, R. L. (1980) *Anorexia Nervosa*, Harmondsworth, Penguin.

Penfold, P. S. and Walker, G. A. (1983) *Women and the Psychiatric Paradox*, Eden Press.

Petchesky, R. P. (1986) *Abortion and Women's Choice: The State, Sexuality and Reproductive Freedom*, London, Verso.

Petchesky, R. P. (1987) 'Foetal images: the power of visual culture in the politics of reproduction', in M. Stanworth (ed.) *Reproductive Technologies: Gender, Motherhood and Medicine*, Cambridge, Polity.

Polhemus, T. (1978) *Social Aspects of the Human Body*, Harmondsworth, Penguin.

Power, E. (1973) *Medieval Women*, Cambridge, Cambridge University Press.

Rich, A. (1980) *On Lies, Secrets and Silence: Selected Prose 1966–1978*, London, Virago.

Roche, L. (1984) *Glutton for Punishment*, London, Pan.

Rothman, B. K. (1986) *The Tentative Pregnancy*, Viking.

Rowbotham, S. (1977) *Hidden from History*, London, Pluto.

Rowbotham, S. (1980) 'The trouble with "patriarchy"', *New Statesman*, 1 Feb.

Russell, D. E. H. (1975) *The Politics of Rape: The Victim's Perspective*, Stein & Day.

Russell, G. F. M. (1977) 'General management of anorexia nervosa and difficulties in assessing the efficacy of treatment', in R. A. Vigersky (ed.) *Anorexia Nervosa*, Raven Press.

Sage, L. (1986) 'Unholy ecstasies', *Observer*, 9 Feb.

Sahlins, M. (1977) *The Use and Abuse of Biology*, London, Tavistock.

Satow, M. (1987) 'Translating realities', in British Sociological Association Equality of the Sexes Committee, 'Proceedings of the workshop on women and research', Nov.

Sayers, J. (1982) *Biological Politics*, London, Tavistock.

Sayers, J. (1987) 'Melanie Klein, psychoanalysis and feminism', *Feminist Review*, 25.

Scull, A. (ed.) (1981) *Madhouses, Mad-doctors, and Madmen: The Social History of Psychiatry in the Victorian Era*, London, Athlone.

Segal, L. (1987) *Is the Future Female? Troubled Thoughts on Contemporary Feminism*, London, Virago.

Showalter, E. (1981) 'Victorian women and insanity', in A. Scull (ed.) *Madhouses, Mad-doctors, and Madmen: The Social History of Psychiatry in the Victorian Era*, London, Athlone.

Skultans, V. (1979) *English Madness: Ideas on Insanity, 1580–1890*, London, Routledge & Kegan Paul.

Slade, R. (1984) *The Anorexia Nervosa Reference Book: Direct and Clear Answers to Everyone's Questions*, New York, Harper & Rowe,

Smith, J. (1978) 'Robert of Arbrissel: procurator mulierum', in D. Baker (ed.) *Medieval Women*, Oxford, Blackwell.

Smith-Rosenberg, C. (1972) 'The hysterical woman', *Social Research*, 39.

Southern, R. W. (1970) *Western Society and the Church in the Middle Ages*, Harmondsworth, Penguin.

Spender, D. (1980) *Man Made Language*, London, Routledge & Kegan Paul.

Spender, D. (ed.) (1983) *Feminist Theorists*, London, Women's Press.

Stannard, U. (1971) 'The mask of beauty', in V. Gornick and B. K. Moran (eds) *Women in Sexist Society*, New York, Basic Books.

Stephens, E. (1976) 'Making changes, making love', *Spare Rib*, 48.

Swartz, L. (1985) 'Is thin a feminist issue?', *Women's Studies International Forum*, Nov.

Thompson, S. (1978) 'The problem of Cistercian nuns in the twelfth and early thirteenth centuries', in D. Baker (ed.) *Medieval Women*, Oxford, Blackwell.

Tickner, L. (1976) 'Fashionable bondage', *Spare Rib*, 47.

Turner, B. S. (1982) 'The discourse of diet', *Theory, Culture & Society*, 1 (1).

Turner, B. S. (1984) *The Body and Society*, Oxford, Blackwell.

Twigg, J. (1983) 'Vegetarianism and the meanings of meat', in A. Murcott (ed.) *The Sociology of Food and Eating*, Aldershot, Gower.

Valverde, M. (1985) *Sex, Power and Pleasure*, Women's Press (Canada).

Vigersky, R. A. (ed.) (1977) *Anorexia Nervosa: A Monograph of the National Institute of Child Health and Human Development*, Raven Press.

Vincent, S. (1984) 'A man cannot rape his wife . . .', *Cosmopolitan*, January.

Warde-Jouve, N. (1984) *The Street-cleaner*, London, Marion Boyars.

Waugh, D. (1988) 'Starving for attention?', *Cosmopolitan*, March.

Weeks, J. (1986) *Sexuality*, London, Tavistock.

Wellbourne, J. and Purgold, J. (1984) *The Eating Sickness: Anorexia, Bulimia and the Myth of Suicide by Slimming*, Brighton, Harvester.

Wilkinson, H. (1984) *Puppet on a String: A Young Girl's Fight to Survive Anorexia Nervosa*, London, Hodder & Stoughton.

Williamson, J. (1985) *Consuming Passions: The Politics and Images of Popular Culture*, London, Marion Boyars.

Willis, E. (1984a) 'Abortion: is a woman a person?', in A. Snitow, S. Stansell and S. Thompson (eds) *Desire: The Politics of Sexuality*, London, Virago.

Willis, E. (1984b) 'Feminism, moralism and pornography', in A. Snitow, S. Stansell and S. Thompson (eds) *Desire: The Politics of Sexuality*, London, Virago.

Zaner, R. (1971) *The Problem of Embodiment: Some Contributions to a Phenomenology of the Body*, Nijhoff.

Name index

Subject index

abortion 161–7

anorexia: and asceticism 20–3, 66, 74; biological explanations 35–8, 44, 198–9; and class 4, 20, 252–3, 255, 256; discovery of 13, 17–23; familial explanations 24–5, 38–44, 45–6, 197–200, 253; feminist explanations 52–87; and mothers 39–40, 54–64, 82–6, 197–200; psychological explanations 24–7, 38–44, 45–9, 70; social explanations 34–6

Anorexic Aid 8, 221

anorexic bodies 2–6, 194–6, 209, 237–44, 246, 248–9, 250, 252

anorexic thinking 35–8, 44–5, 223, 230

appetite 212–13; control by 223–4, 233–4, 239, 241–2, 244–6, 250–1; control of 107, 194, 203–6, 241–3, 247–8, 250–2; as dangerous 195, 207–9, 213; as insatiable 101–2, 107–9, 194–5, 206–7, 227, 249–50; as natural 28, 83–4, 98, 234

asceticism 124–6, 128–9, 140, 197

assertiveness 34, 40

beauty 156, 160, 173–8, 204

bingeing 218, 226, 228–35, 242, 250, 293

body, the: bourgeois concept of 42–4, 113–14, 118, 137–57, 173, 248–9; feudal concept of 44, 113, 119–37, 157; as metaphor 115–16, 118, 141–2, 197, 209; and mind 140–1, 149–52; as natural phenomenon 116–19, 147, 153; oppositional concepts 113, 119, 130–7, 139, 143, 147, 156–7; as a social construction 2–3, 6, 44, 50, 72, 83–4, 113–19, 141, 153, 158–9; and soul 124–6, 128–9

boundaries 65, 78; around the body 84, 115–16, 132–6, 139–40, 150, 191; between self and environment 72, 81, 150–1

bourgeois culture 138, 148, 155, 254, 257

bourgeois individualism 44, 63, 85, 138, 252–3

bulimia 106–8, 197, 228–31, 234, 242

capitalism 137–8, 140, 142–3, 148, 155, 158

castration 144–6, 179

childhood 22, 27

clitoridectomy 114–15

control: by anorexia 238–43, 246; by the body 239, 241, 243; of the body 155–6, 161–6, 248, 193–4, 201; loss of 224–6, 228–35, 245; by others 223–4, 228, 230–1, 238, 244–6; of